Exploring Herbs

DIABETES MELLITUS

Priya Rao

INTRODUCTION

Introduction

India produces largest praprtion of medicnal herbs and is understood as installation of the planet. These herbs are used for hundreds of years, in one type or different, beneath the various systems of drugs like Siddha , Unani and therefore the most significant Ayurveda.

The quest for a healthier lifestyle has made people to recognize the healing power of these medicinal herbs again. Traditional medicines were the sole approach to health for each and every country, and have been passed on from generation to this day Herbal remedies work with no unpleasant side effects found in modern medicines.

1.1 Medicine

The "traditional medicine" is the only way of protecting and restoring health that existed scienc ancient time. Traditional medicines were the sole approach to health for each and every country, and have been passed on from generation to this day.

The World Health Organization outlined traditional drugs, as comprising therapeutic practices that are breathing, typically for many years, before the event and development of synthetic drugs and still in use **(WHO, 1991)**.

1.2 Herbal Medicine

As per WHO -"Any plant and its parts containing any substance which can be used therapeutically, or used as raw material for drug/ Chemical synthesis is categorized as herbal medicine."

It has been described as the oldest form of therapy practiced by humans today, with archaeological evidence of medicinal use of herbs dating back to 60,000 years. Herbal medicines often complement predictable treatments, providing safe as well as well tolerated remedies for chronic illness. The crude drugs which includes plant, animal or mineral origin, is like an instrumental aid to a physician, where the art and skill of formulation ensures that poisonous drug could be transformed into vary safe and effective drug **(Rangari V.D. 2002)**.

INTRODUCTION

India has a wealthy ancestry of science of plants based on drugs both for use in remedial and preventive medicine. All the rich sources of plant material and their knowledge has led Indian scientists to discover challenging aspects of crude drugs for pharmaceutical & medicinal uses, in search for new and more potent drugs. Plant drugs offer marked therapeutic values and negligible side effects, economy and easy availability **(Ansari S.H 1998).**

The substantial scientific work that has been skilled in recent years in the field of pharmaceuticals and natural products has significantly revolutionized the entire concept. This has rekindled the interest in the continued and extensive use of plant products. In spite of so much potential and scope of future development of herbal drugs, we have not achieved benefit of even 2% of total flora provided by nature. Therefore, future of herbal drugs depends upon the maintenance of quality control, therapeutic credibility and proper research funding and sincere commitment to research on plant drugs and remedies.

Herbal medicines, primarily used by developing countries for primary health care. They need stood the take a look at of your time for his or her safety, efficacy, cultural acceptableness and lesser or no aspect effects. Herbals are used for health care through-out the globe since the earliest days of humans, are frequently used nowdays, and recognition of their clinical, pharmaceutical and economic values that are still growing.

1.2.1 Merits of Herbal Medicine

Herbal remedies are effective, easily available and cheap. The future trend is more towards everything "NATURAL" and the four distinct areas where "NATURAL" is given preference are:-

- **Environment:** grow more plants, conservation of forests and creation of green belt to avoid environmental pollution.
- **Food:** maximum stress on meals containing fresh vegetables.
- **Cosmetics:** Herbal creams, Shampoos, Toiletries are becoming much more popular.

INTRODUCTION

> **Medicines:** Herbal medicines have growing interest and concern to millions of people. There are apparent signs of rejuvenation of interest in therapeutically useful plants.

1.2.2 The Reason for Popularity of Herbal Medicines

> They stood the take a look at for his or her safety and efficacy

> Active constituents in these medicines have physiological effectin living flora and they're compatible with body.

> Ancient literature additionally mentions herbal medicines for age connected diseases specifically diabetes, wounds, immune and liver disorders etc.

1.3 Regulation Of Issues For Traditional Medicines

Traditional drugs could be a broad term encompassing health practices, approaches, data and beliefs that incorporate flavouring, animal and mineral primarily based medicines, religious therapies, manual techniques and exercises, applied singularly or together to treat, diagnose and forestall sicknesses or maintain well-being **(W.H.O. 2004)**. nowadays though, there has been plenty of interest within the ancient drugs for its potential contribution to health care, there ar issues regarding the standard drugs for effectivity, safety and quality. A recent W.H.O. fact sheet comments "Unregulated or inappropriate use of traditional medicines and practices can have negative or dangerous effects." Our National Policy (2001) on Indian Systems of Medicine includes issues such as drug standards, regulations, enforcement and focuses the research agenda on clinical trials, pharmacology, toxicology and drug standardization. In recent years, several regulatory guidelines are available in the area of herbal medicines.

1.4. Safety or adverse effects of Herbal medicine.

Inappropriate formulation, adulteration, or less understanding of drug and plant interactions may lead to adverse reactions that are sometimes life threatening or very lethal." A number of herbs are unit thought to be possible to cause aspect effects. moreover, " inappropriate formulation, adulteration, or less understanding of drug and plant interactions might result in adverse reactions that are life threatening or terriblydeadly

INTRODUCTION

"correct single blind or double-blind clinical trials are unitrequiredto work out the security and efficaciousness of every plant before they'll be counseled for medical use. Though several shoppers believe that flavorer medicines area unit safe as a result of they're "natural", flavorer medicines and artificial medication might move, and as a results of interaction cause toxicity to the patient. Herbal medicines may be seriously contaminated, and herbal medicines with none established efficaciousness parameter, might unwittingly be wont to replace medicines that do have substantiated efficaciousness. Standardization of purity and indefinite quantity isn't mandated within the North American country, however same merchandisecreated to identical specification might disagree as a results of organic chemistry variations among identical species of plant. medicative Plants have a robust defensive measure mechanisms against predators that may have deadly or adverse effects on humans being. There are some samples of extremely hepatotoxic herbs that embrace poison woody plant and hemlock. These product cannot marketed in public as herbs, as a result of the risks of life threatening result area unitrenowned are renowned, partdue to a protracted ancient and colourful history in Europe, related to"sorcery", "magic" and intrigue. Widespread use of herbs isn'treported to possess non adverse reactions. On rare occasions serious untoward results are joined to herb consumption. a serious case of metal depletion has been attributed to chronic bodily process of licorice, and since of this skilled herbalists/scientist avoid the utilization of licorice once they recognized this risk. A number of studies are unit accessible on the security of herbs for pregnant girls, and one amongst that study found that use of other and complementary medicines are unitrelated to a half-hour lower current gestation and nativity rate throughout fertility treatment. Samples of flavorer treatments that possible cause-effect relationships with adverse events embrace poisonous plant, that is usually a de jure restricted herb. Ayurvedic remedies, Chinese herb mixtures comfrey, herbs containing suresubshrub flavonoids, guar gum, pennyroyal and liquorice root, are unit samples of herbs with a high degree of confidence of a risk and future adverse effects is declared. Ginseng, that is less-traveled among herbalists attributable to this reason, the vulnerable herb species like shrub, milk weed, goldenseal, instead that herbalists typically advise and really some seldom use plant species , buckthorn bark and berry, kava, aloe vera juice, chittam bark bark, valerian, scrub palmetto, which is totally restricted within the world organization.

INTRODUCTION

For example, acute low pressure might result from the mix of associate in Nursing favorers remedy that lowers pressure in conjunction with ethical drug that has identical outcome. A number of herb might amplify the results of anticoagulants. Sure herbs in addition as common fruit move with hemoprotein P450, associate in nursing catalyst essential to drug metabolism.

1.5 Standards and Quality Control of Herbal Medicine.

The issue of regulation is a locality of continuous role within the USA and EU . At one end, some scientist/herbalists maintain that ancient remedies have a really long history of use, Associate don't need any level of safety testing as xenobiotics or single ingredients in an by artificial mean stargeted type. In different facet of frame ,some others square measure in favor of lawfully enforced safety testing, quality standards, and prescription by a professional person. Within which some skilled person establishment have opinions statements line for a class of rule and regulation for the herbal product. Whereas others consider the requirement for additional quality testing customary however believe that to be managed internally while not government intervention. Position of any seasoning ingredients disagree by in step with the origin of country. At the Europe, herbal medicines measure currently synchronic to a lower place the eudirective on ancient seasoning healthful product. In the u. s., most herbal remedies measure regulated as dietary supplements by the Food and Drug Administration(USFDA). Producer of those product falling into this class don't seem to be needed to prove the protection or effectuality of their product; although the office could with drawa product from sale if found harmful. The industry's largest trade association named National nutritionary Foods Association, has running a program from 2002, examining closely to the merchandise and producing conditions of their member firms, and supply them the proper to show the GMP (Good producing Practices) seal of approval on their product. Some herbs, like Cannabis, square measure fully illegal in most countries. Since 2004, the sale of bush as dietary supplement is prohibited within the U. S. by the Food and Drug Administration **(Goldman P, 2001).**

INTRODUCTION

1.6 Standardization of Herbal Medicines

All artificial medication are ready victimization pure artificial materials; duplicable producing techniques and acceptable chemical assay of the medication, that are given in Pharmacopoeias having adequate internal control. In distinction, seasoning medicines of plant origin are unit vulnerable to contamination, deterioration and variation in compositions, issues for internal control and testing of those herbal medication and therefore improper standardized product. Standardization of that herbal product is an important measuring for making certain the standard management of the herbal medication. Many factors like atmosphere, genetic strategies of cultivation, collection, preparation, storage etc., have an effect on the standard of the herbal medication. The assemblage standards in Ayurvedic Pharmacopoeia of Republic of India aren't adequate enough to confirm the standard of plant materials and also the later product. Therefore, Chemical strategies, Instrumental strategies and Thin Layer chromatographical analysis would verify the right quality of plants materials. Therefore, in-house specifications for the plant materials ought to be developed to modify the standard management of herbal product. Standardization is employed to explain all measures, that are unit throughout the production method and internal control resulting in a duplicable quality. Standardization expression conjointly encompasses the whole field of study from birth of a plant to its clinical application**(Werner, 2000).**

Standardization is that the basic prerequisite for consistent effectiveness of herbal medicative product. No matter the question of whether or not the active constituents of associate herbal drugare better-known or not, each producing method leading to associate herbal medicative product must be submitted for standardization.

This standardization includes standards about the subsequent (**Stuttgart 2003**):

- ➤ The herbal drug raw materials.
- ➤ The extraction solvent
- ➤ The production method.
- ➤ In method controls.
- ➤ The herbal drug preparation.

INTRODUCTION

The constituents of Standardized herbal preparations are classified into 3 categories:
1. Therapeutically active constituents: with chemicals outlined substances or teams of drugs, which, in associate isolated state, exert identical or similar therapeutic result, because the total extract.

2. Active constituents: with chemical ubstances or teams of drugs that, in associate isolated state, don't exert identical therapeutic result as a complete extract, however that are unit accepted to contribute to the therapeutic activity of the seasoning drug preparation.
3. Markers: with chemical substances or teams of drugs, that solely serve analytical functions.

a) Characteristic markers: these area unit markers appropriate for standardization of medicative plants (e.g. batch to batch control)
b) Ubiquitous marker: occur ubiquitously in plants, appropriate for assay (e.g. batch to batch control).

1.6.1 Quality Control Of Herbs And Extracts

There are variations between preparations and with chemicals synthesized product, the fundamental quality needs are constant, that is, identity, purity and content determination, the standards permanently producing follow (WHO Technical Reports Series, No. 863, 1996). Internal control begins at the amount of the beginning material. The stuffis that the most vital demand within the producing of herbal healthful product. Plants constituents ar irregular as a result of their composition could also be influenced by multiple factors, for instance, origin, growth, harvesting, drying and storage conditions. By creating use of cultivated plants, causes of variability could also be eliminated.

Adulterations should be taken into thoughtoncethe fabric is purchased from industrial sources. Consistent quality for product of seasoner origin willsolely be assured if the beginning materials are outlined in an exceedingly rigorous and careful manner. Besides biology identification of the stuff used, the exclusion or limitation of impurities like alternative plant components or foreign matter, microorganisms, and their metabolites is very important.

INTRODUCTION

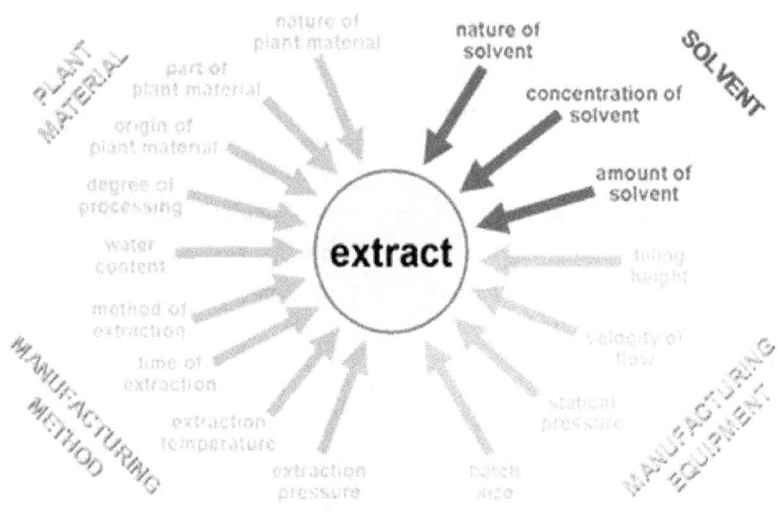

Figure 1.1: Variables to be Managed for the Preparation of an identical Extract

1.6.2 Pharmacopeial standards

The Pharmacopeial standards in Ayurvedic assemblage of Asian nationdon't seem to been enough to confirm the standard of plant materials, since the materials received within theproducing premises don't seem to be in a very condition that effective microscopic examinations are often done. Therefore, varied analysis, Instrumentation analysis and Thin Layer analysis would verify the correct quality of plant materials. For this, In house specifications for the plant materials ought to be developed to changethe standardmanagement Chemist to verify and approve the materials (**Stuttgart,2003**).The in house specifications ought to cowl the subsequent :-

i) Chemical assay: Specific assay for active principles, e.g. total alkaloids, resins, essential oil, glycosides, saponins, tannins, etc square measuredole out by completely different chemical strategies.

ii) Instrumental analysis: Major active constituents square measure quantified by instrument (HPLC/HPTLC/GC) or Spectrophotometrical strategies.

iii) Extractive values: Alcohol and water – soluble extractive values provide a concept regarding the standard of herb.

iv) Ash values: Total ash, Acid insoluble and Water soluble ash square measure useful in standardizing the herbs.

v) Foreign matter: Any foreign matter apart from the required half together with insects, rodents oranimal waste shouldn't be gift.

vi) Microbial contamination: Herbs ought to be clean and will be free from any pathogens, bacteria, moulds or plant. If heating isn't concerned within the production method, herbs ought to be properly sterilized by chemical compound or electromagnetic radiation.

vii) Quantitative microscopy: Just in case of fine herbs, it's generally troublesome to differentiate between adulterant and real plant. Quantitative microscopical techniques facilitate to differentiate allied species.

viii) Herbicide/pesticide residues: correct testing procedures ought to be developed in order that these residues square measure well at intervals limits.

INTRODUCTION

1.6.3 Who Guidelines For Quality Control Of Herbal Materials

- Sampling.
- Macroscopic and microscopic analysis.
- Thin layer activity analysis.
- Arsenic and significant metals content.
- Microbial load and absence of pathogens.
- Pesticide residues.
- Extractable matter.
- Ash content.
- Foreign matter.
- Volatile oil content.
- Hemolytic activity.
- Foaming index.
- Tannin content.
- Bitter value.

1.7   Stability Testing Of Herbal Medicines

Stability testing is necessary to ensure that the product is of acceptable quality throughout its entire storage period. With the help of modern analytical techniques like spectrophotometry, HPLC, HPTLC and by employing proper guidelines it is possible to generate a sound stability data of herbal products and forecast their shelf-life, which helps in improving global acceptability of herbal products **(Kathrin *et al.*, 2003)**.

1.8   Regulatory Status Of Herbal Medcines

The legal situation of herbal medicines varies from country to country. Developing countries have folk knowledge of herbs and their use in traditional medicine is wide spread. But, these countries have any legislative criteria to include herbal medicines in drug legislation **(Sukhdev *et al.*, 2008)**. Regulatory requirements for herbal medicines are necessary to ensure the safety, efficacy and quality and to support specific indications, through scientific and clinical evidences **(Mukherjee, 2006)**.

INTRODUCTION

1.9 Diabetes

Diabetes mellitus is a metabolic disorder occurs due to deficiency or failure of normal action of insulin **(Asakawa *et al.*, 2006)**.

1.9.1 Types of Diabetes

Diabetes mellitus is classified intofollowing categories:

Insulin-Dependent Diabetes (Type 1)

Insulin deficiency produced due to selective β cell destruction, in this insulin therapy is essential. It is due to immune and idiopathic causes.

Noninsulin-Dependent Diabetes (Type 2)

This is a multifactorial metabolic disorder characterized by hyperglycemia due to a defective insulin secretion or insulin resistance or reduced insulin sensitivity. It is related to disease state, environmental impact and food habit.

Gestational Diabetes Mellitus (Type 3)

Insulin resistance developed due to placenta and placental hormones which lead to abnormal glucose in pregnancy.

Neonatal diabetes mellitus

Due to defects in chromosome in first trimester of pregnancy blood glucose level is disturbed. **(Craig et al 2009).**

Mitochondrial diabetes

Beta-cell failure occurs, sensorineural deafnes is associated with it.

Cystic fibrosis related diabetes

It is due to infections and medications, and impaired glucose tolerance developed .

INTRODUCTION

1.9.2 Prevalence and incidence of diabetes mellitus

According to the WHO, more than 245 million people suffering with diabetes and up to 2025 it is more than 380 million. India has the world's largest diabetes population with estimated 35 million patient and known as "Capital of diabetes mellitus" **(Patel *et al.*, 2009)**. Eldery population are more affected by diabetes. Females are more susseptable than male. **(Trout and Teff, 2004)**.

1.9.3 Pathology of Diabetes mellitus

It causes hyperglycemia where blood sugar level is elevated above 120 mg/dl, normal blood glucose level being 80-120 mg/dl. It is referred to glycosuria in presence of glucose in urine. The blood glucose levels in diabetic conditions are above 180 mg/dl. In addition, due to lack of insulin the transport of glucose into the tissue is decreased (though the blood glucose levels may be high) and hence, the liver increases the oxidation of fatty acids to satisfy energy requirements, which also increases Acetyl Co-A production. All this leads to a decrease in blood pH, which leads to ketoacidosis.

1.9.4 Complication of Diabetes

Acute complications of diabetes is ketoacidosis, which finally can produce coma **(Boon *et al.*, 2006)**. Diabetic retinopathy, neuropathy and nephropathy are complication along with gastrointestinal problems, hardening of blood vessels and stroke (**Raghuram *et al.*, 2003)**.

1.9.5 Diagnosis of Diabetes

Following measures to be adopted for this

(A) Glucose level in blood

. In a normal individualthe FBG 100 mg/dl and post-meal value up to140 mg/dl and their diagnostic interpretation **(American Diabetes Association, 1998) (Table 1.2)**.

INTRODUCTION

Table 1.1 : Glucose level as a diagnostic tool in diabetes

Conditions	Normal	Pre-diabetic	Diabetic
Fasting	Less than 100	101-125	More than 126
2 h Post meal	Less than 140	140-199	More than 200

If 2 hours post meal glucose is more than 140 but less than 200 mg/dl it is known as impaired glucose tolerance. Both the above conditions indicate high possibility of diabetes in the future.

(B)   Oral glucose tolerance test (OGTT)

If case of problems in diagnosis, the OGTT is advised. Where fasting blood glucose sample is tested, but instead of food for post-meal test 82.5 gm of glucose (equivalent to 75 gm. anhydrous glucose) mixed in one glass of water and gives to subject. Moreover the diagnostic interpretation of OGTT is carried out, after 2 hours of glucose consumptions.

1.10   Current Preventative Strategies for Diabetes mellitus

Although diabetes is not curable, but it is possible to lead a healthy normal life by keeping glucose level under control. Diabetes is a metabolic syndrome and glucose disorder is a part of it. The other problems associated with this disorder are high blood pressure, high cholesterol etc.

Lifestyle Modifications for managing the diabetes may involve reduction in body weight, enhanced physical activity, increased dietary fibers, limited carbohydrate intake and quitting smoking. Following steps can be taken

- Regular exercise
- Diet management
- Life style changes
- Oral medication and
- Insulin

INTRODUCTION

If secretion of hypoglycaemic agent from the exocrine gland decreases then oral medication are given to extend the secretion of hypoglycaemic agent. Even once the patients are on oral medication they ought to follow strict diet management and regular exercise schedule. If followed, diet management and exercise makes antidiabetic drug tablets/drugs simpler. If the exocrine gland beta-cells range is incredibly less there is need of external hypoglycaemic agent. (Figure 1.2).

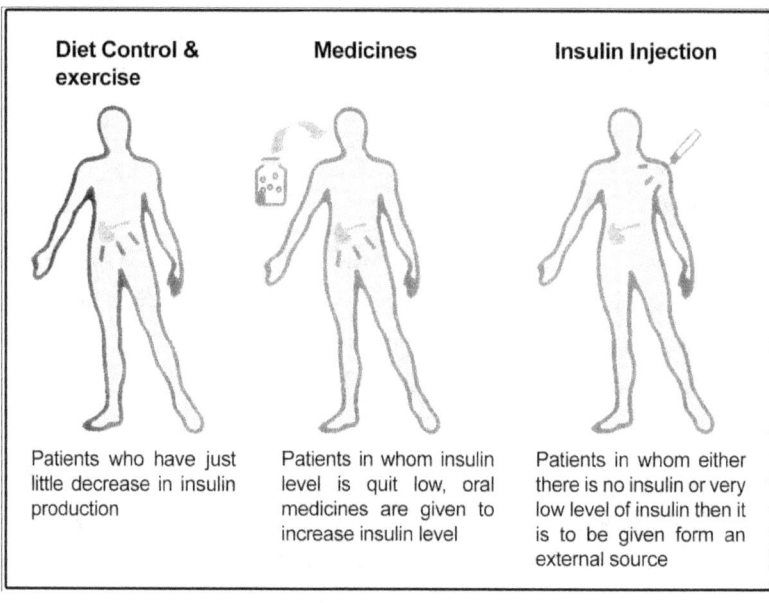

Figure 1.2 : The controlling regimen of diabetes

INTRODUCTION

1.10.1 Synthetic Antidiabetic Drugs

Many class of synthetic drugs such as Sulfonylurea, Meglitinides, Biguanides, Thiazolidinediones, Alpha glucosidase inhibitors, Amylin analogue, Incretin mimetic, DPP-4 inhibitors are available for diabetes **(Levobitz, 2004).**

Limitations, side effects and drawbacks of synthetic drugs: (Dey *et al.*, 2002).

- development of resistance
- lack of responsiveness
- liver toxicity;
- heart diseases,
- increase the body weight
- bloating, flatulence, diarrhea
- abdominal discomfort and pain

1.10.2 Herbal Treatment for diabetes

The knowledge of diabetes existed with the Indians since prehistoric age. Herbal formulations are used by a majority of population throughout the world, since ancient time. **(Eddouks *et al.*, 2004).** Traditionally above 1200 plants are used for this **(Kesari *et al.*, 2007).** Antihyperglycemic effect of several plant extracts or formulations has been confirmed. as per **Feshani et al 2011 and Pareek et al 2009** plants and their formulations (indigenous remedies) are used for diabetes.

1.10.3 Advance therapeutic approaches to preserve islets mass in Type-2 diabetes

Progressive reductions in β-cell mass contribute considerably to the pathological process of Type-2 diabetes. a significant goal of it's analysis is to revive the β-cell mass that's generally lost throughout the natural progression of Type-2 diabetes. The glucagons-like peptide-1 receptor agonists, and related peptides such as gastric inhibitory polypeptide are suggested to preserve and/or restore functional β-cell mass in diabetics (Table 1.2).

Table 1.2 : Agents that increase / preserve β-cell mass

Stimulators of β-cell proliferation or neogenesis	**Inhibitors of β-cell death**
Prolactin	Glucagons-like peptide-1 receptor
Betacellulin	Gastric inhibitory polypeptide
Glucagons-like peptide-1 receptor	Dipeptidyl-peptidase-IV
Dipeptidyl-peptidase-IV	Hepatocyte growth factors
Gastric inhibitory polypeptide	Insulin-like growth factors
Thiazolidinediones	Parathyroid hormone-related peptide
Hepatocyte growth factor	
Human placental lactogen	
Insulin-like factors	
Parathyroid hormone-related peptide	
Growth hormone insulin-like growth factors	

INTRODUCTION

1.11 Animal Models in Type–2 Diabetes Research

A wide range of animal models are used for diabetes (Srinivasan *et al.* 2007 and Karalee *et al.*, 2001).

Table 1.3: Diabetogenic agents for induction of diabetes

Agents	Species	Dose's (mg/kg)
Alloxan	Rat	40-200
	Mice	50-200
	Rabbit	100-150
	Dog	50-75
Streptozotocin	Rat	36-65
	Mice	100-200
	Dog	20-30
	Hamster	50
	Pig	100-500
Dehydro ascorbic acid	Rat	650 mg/kg three days
Dehydro isoascorbic acid	Rat	1.5mg/kg
Dehydrogluco ascorbic acid	Rat	3.5 to 3.9g/kg
Methyl alloxan	Rat	53 mg/kg
Ethyl alloxan	Rat	50-130mg/kg
Oxine and dithizone	Rabbit	50mg/kg
Sodium diethyldithio-carbonate	Rabbit	0.5 to 1g/kg
Potassium xanthate	Rabbit	200-350mg/kg
Uric acid	Rabbit	1g/kg

INTRODUCTION

1.12 : Objective of research

        Diabetes mellitus characterized by hyperglycemia effective cure for which is unavailable. Exercise, chemotherapy and diet only manages it. The synthetic drugs used for diabetes are too expensive and also have undesirable side effects or contraindications. Search of effective antidiabetic agents is still continuing. The WHO also suggested use of plants/plant drived product as drugs. And the same stands true for diabetes. fortunately our country has been blessed with a large treasure of plant possessing antidiabetic activity. But due to lack of exhaustive research work till date no effective formulation for diabetes could be developed. Similarly no single drug has been found to control diabetes. On the basis of literature survey, market survey and consulting from traditional drug practitioners plants selected for study with the objective of developing potential antidiabetic formulation.

1.13   Plan of Works

- Literature Survey.
- Identification, collection, drying, powdering of plant materials for extraction
- Organoleptic characterization
- Phytochemical screening
- Extraction
- In vitro and in vivo antidiabetic screening of different extracts
- Selection of extracts with better antidiabetic activity
- Preparation of fractions and in vivo antidiabetic screening of different fractions
- Selection of fractions with better antidiabetic activity
- Development of antidiabetic formulation
- its comparison with allopathic standard and available marketed herbal formulation

INTRODUCTION

Details of *in vivo* study:

- Estimation of glucose concentration
    - Fasting blood glucose
    - oral glucose tolerance test determination
- Estimation of blood profile
    - total haemoglobin content
    - albumin and other protein content
- Estimation of lipid profile
    - Plasma triglycerides
    - Serum cholesterol
    - L.D.L.
    - H.D.L.
- Estimation of enzymes activity
- Histopathological studies

REVIEW OF LITERATURE

2.1 Introduction

Since time immamorial, plants have used as rich source of medicine. In Atharv-Veda and Charak and Sushrut Samhita (100-500 BC) detailed descriptions of over 700 herbs are given. Diabetes mellitus is caused by the abnormality or disfunction of carbohydrate metabolism. Antihyperglycemic effect of several plant extracts or formulations has been confirme. As per ancient literature, more than 800 plants are reported to have antidiabetic properties. Some plants having hypoglycemic and/or antihyperglycemic potential are as follows **(Devaliya and Shirsat, 2017; Table2. 1).**

Table 2. 1: Plants having hypoglycemic and/or antihyperglycemic or antidiabetic potential

Botanical Name	Family	Mode of action
Abelmoschus moschatus Medik	Malvaceae	Antidiabetic activity
Abies pindrow	Pinaceae	Insulin secretagogue activity
Abroma augusta	Sterculiaceae	Hypoglycemic activity
Abrus precatorius L.	Fabaceae	Antidiabetic activity
Acacia arabica Babul / Indian Gum	Leguminosae	Insulin secretagogue activity
Achiliea santolina	Asteraceae	Hypoglycemic and antioxidant activity
Achyranthus aspera	Amaranthaceae	Hypoglycemic activity
Achyrocline satureioides	Asteraceae	Hypoglycemic and antioxidant activity,
Aconitum carmichaelii	Ranunculaceae	Antidiabetic activity
Acosmium panamense (Benth.)	Leguminosae	Lowers the plasma glucose levels
Adhatoda vasica Nees	Acanthaceae	Antidiabetic activity
Aegle marmelos Bael/Golden apple	Rutaceae	Increases utilization of glucose or by Insulin secretagogue activity

REVIEW OF LITERATURE

Aerva lanata (L.) Sunny khur.	Amaranthaceae	Its alcohol extract reduced blood sugar level To be continue..................
Agrimony eupatoria	Rosaceae	Insulin releasing activity
Agrimonia pilosa	Rosaceae	Hypoglycemic and Antidiabetic activity
Allium cepa ,Pyaj	Liliaceae	hypoglycemic and hypocholesterolemic effect; anti-diabetic and anti-hyperlipidemic
Allium sativum (L.) (*Alliaceae*) Lahasun,	Liliaceae	Hypoglycemic and Antidiabetic activity; It increases serum insulin level and improves glucose tolerance
Aloe barbadensis	Liliaceae	Stimulating synthes is and/or release of insulin
Aloe vera . Ghee Kunwar / Kumar pantha	Liliaceae	Antidiabetic activity
Anacardium occidentale Linn.	Anacardiaceae	Antidiabetic activity
Andrographis lineate Nees	Acanthaceae	Control the blood sugar level
Andrograhis paniculata, Kalmegh	Acanthaceae	glucose utilization increased
Annona muricata Linn. , soursop	Annonaceae	prevents β cells degeneration
Annona squamosa Sitafal /Sugar apple / Custard apple	Annonaceae	Hypoglycemic and antihyperglycemic activities;
Aralia elata	Araliaceae,	hypoglycemic activity is mediated through inhibition of aldose reductase activity
Areca catechu (L.) Supari/ Betel nut	Arecaceae	Subcutaneous administration of its alkaloid fraction have hypoglycemic effect; Arecoline, isolated from its nuts, reported to have hypoglycemic activity
Artemosia dracunculus L. Dragon herb	Asteraceae	Hypoglycemic action

REVIEW OF LITERATURE

Artemisia pallens Davana	Compositae	Antihyperglycemic activity
Artemisia sphaerocephala Worm wood	Asteraceae	Hypoglycemic and Antidiabetic activity
Astragalus propinquus Schischkin	Leguminosae	Decreases the blood glucose
Averrhoa bilimbi	Oxalidaceae	Increases serum insulin level
Azadirachta indica Neem	Meliaceae	Having glycogenolytic effect
Barleria lupulina Lind/ Snake bush	Acanthaceae	methanol extract of aerial parts showed hyperglycemic activity
Bauhinia forficata	Caesalpinaceae	Hypoglycemic and Antidiabetic activity
Beta vulgaris Chukander / Garden beet	Chenopodiaceae	Reducing blood glucose level by regeneration of ß cells
Bidens pilosa	Compositae	Reducing blood glucose level
Biophytum sensitivum (L.) DC Lajjalu /Life plant	. (*Oxalidaceae*)	antihyperglycemic ; an insulinotropic effect
Bixa orellana	Bixaceae	plasma insulin increased
Boerhaavia diffusa Punarnava/Red hogweed	Nyctaginaceae	hexokinase and glucose-6-phosphatase activity incresed
Bougainvillea spectabilis	Nyctaginaceae	antihyperglycemic action
Bombax ceiba (L) Semul / Red silk cotton tree .	Bombacaceae	Hypoglycemic activity
Brassica juncea	Cruciferae	Food adjuvants for diabetic patients
Brassica nigra	Brassicaceae	Reduce serum glucose and serum lipids; stimulate insulin release
Bridelia ndellensis Beille.	Euphorbiaceae	stimulate of islets cells and requires functional β-cells for its action
Butea monosperma Bastard	Fabaceae	Hypoglycemic activity

REVIEW OF LITERATURE

teak/Flame of the Forest		
Caesalpinia bonducella Kantkarej/ Kantikaranja/ Fever nut	Cesalpinaceae	Free radicle scavenging activity; ethanol and aqueous extract produced significant antihyperglycemic effect
Cajanus cajan (L) Millsp. Tuvar/ Red gram	Fabaceae	Antihyperglycemic action
Camellia sinensis Tea	Theaceae	hot water extract significantly reduced the blood glucose level; Increasing insulin secretion
Canavalia ensiformis DC. horse bean	Leguminosae	Reduce urinary and blood glucose levels, and also elevated levels of triacylglycerol, ketone bodies and cholesterol
Capparis deciduas Keekar/Karir/Kirir, / Caper	Capparidaceae	Hypoglycemic, antioxidant, hypolipidaemic plant fruit powder hypoglycemia
Capsicum frutescens	Solanaceae	Increased insulin secretion
Carica papaya Papaya	Caricaceae	Hypoglycemic activity
Casearia esculenta Roxb Saptarangi /wild cowrie fruit	Flacourtiaceae	hypolipidemic and antioxidant
Cassia auriculata Tanner's Cassia	Caesalpiniaceae	Decrese blood glucose and lipid
Catharanthus roseus Sadabahar/periwinkle	Apocynaceae	Increasing metabolisation of glucose; regulate the blood sugar level
Chamaemelum nobile (L.)	Asteraceae	Aqueous extract reduces blood glucose level
Cinnamomum zeylanicum Dalchini	Lauraceae	Elevate plasma insulin ; cinnamaldehyde reduce serum glucose and glycosylated hemoglobin
Citrullus colocynthis (L.) Schrad. Indryan/ Bitter apple	Cucurbitaceae	aqueous extract reduce plasma glucose

REVIEW OF LITERATURE

Clausena anisata	Rutaceae	Stimulating secretion of insulin
Coccinia indica Kundru,	*Cucurbitaceae*)	Antilipidemic
Coptis chinensis (*Huanglian*)	Ranunculaceae	potentiates insulin receptor expression in liver and skeletal muscle cells caused regeneration in the damaged pancreas
Coriandrum sativum	Umbelliferae	Decrease blood sugar
Coscinium fenestratum	Menispermaceae	Increasing enzymatic antioxidants
Croton cajucara	Euphorbiaceae	Lowering plasma glucose level
Curcuma longa (L.) Haldi /Turmeric .	*Zingiberaceae*)	Decrease blood sugar
Cyamopsis tetragonoloba	Fabaceae	Reduces blood glucose levels
Cynodon dactylon Pers. Doob	Poaceae	aqueous extract have antidiabetic effects along with hypoglycemic and hypolipidemic effects
Dioscorea dumetorum Pax. (Dioscoreaceae),	Dioscoreaceae	dioscoretine, hasbeen reported to possess hypoglycemic effect
Eclipta alba	Compositae	Decreasing activity of glucose-6phosphatase and fructose-1-6,biphasphatase
Embellica officinalis Gaertn.	Euphorbiaceae	Reducing 5- hydroxymethylfurfural,creatinine albumin level
Enicostemma littorale Chhota Chirata / White-head.	Gentianaceae	Decreasing glycosylated Hb and glucose 6 phosphatase
Eugenia jambolana Jamun	Myrtaceae	Lowering plasma glucose level hypoglycemic and decreased glycosuria, restoring the altered hepatic and skeletal muscle glycogen
Eucalyptus globulus	Myrtaceae	insulin secretogauge

REVIEW OF LITERATURE

Eugenia uniflora (L.) Surinam Cherry / Brazilian	*Myrtaceae*	Antihyperglycemic
Ficus religiosa	Moraceae	Initiating release of insulin
Ficus bengalensis Bargad / Banyan	Moraceae	Rising serum insulin; hot water and ethanol extract of its bark and aerial roots have antidiabetic activity
Ficus hispida Linn. Al, Daduri	(Moraceae),	water-soluble fraction of the alcoholic extract has directperipheral action on β cells
Ficus racemosa Linn. Gular'	*Moraceae*	α-amyrin acetate is antidiabetic
Gentiana olivieri	Gentianaceae	Hypoglycemic, anti-hyperlipidemic
Ginkgo biloba L.	Ginkgoaceae	Hypoglycemic, increases pancreatic beta-cells
Globularia alypum L.	Globulariaceae	Hypoglycemic, increases plasma insulin levels
Gymnema montanum Gurmar	Asclepiadaceae	Antioxidant& antiperoxidative
Gymnema sylvestre Gurmar or Gurmarbooti	Asclepiadaceae	Lowering plasma glucose level
Gentiana olivier.	Gentianaceae	Lowering plasma glucose level
Glycerrhiza glabra, Licorice.	Leguminosae	Lowering plasma glucose level; Glycyrrhizin, isolated from licorice root showed potential antihyperglycemic effect
Glycine max Soya beans	Fabaceae	Hypoglycemic activity
Grewia asiatica Phalsa / Falsa	Malvaceae	anti-hyperglycemic action
Gynura procumbens	Compositae	Hypoglycemic activity

REVIEW OF LITERATURE

Helicteres isora (L.) Marodphalli	*Sterculiaceae*	its bark extract reduces lipids in diabetic rats
Hibiscus rosa sinensis Gudhal/ Shoe flower	Malvaceae	Stimulating insulin secretion from beta cells; ethanol extract lowered the total cholesterol and serum triglycerides
Hintonia latiflora	Rubiaceae	anti-hyperglycemic activity
Hygrophila auriculata Heine	(*Acanthaceae*)	antidiabetic and potent antioxidant
Hypoxis hemerocallidea Fisch. Mey.	Hypoxidaceae	hypoglycemic and Antidiabetic activity
Ipomoea aquatica	Convolvulaceae	Reducing fasting blood sugar level and serum glucose level
Indigofera mysorensis	Fabaceae	ethanol extract have insulin sensitizing property
Ipomoea batata sweet potato	Convolvulaceae	Reducing insulin resistance and blood glucose level; stimulating human immunity
Justicia tranquebarienis L.f.	Acanthaceae	Increasing peripheral glucose consumption and induce insulin secretion
Lactuca indica (L.)Indian Lettuce.	*Asteraceae*	hypoglycemic
Lantana camara (L.) Caturang	Verbenaceae	hypoglycemic effect
Lepidium sativum	Cruciferae	Reducing blood glucose level
Lupinus albus	Fabaceae	Lowering serum glucose level
Lyophyllum decastes Fried chicken mushroom	Lyophyllaceae	Antidiabetic activity
Mangifera indica	Anacardiaceae	Reduction of intestinal absorption of glucose

REVIEW OF LITERATURE

Aam / Mango		
Memecylon umbellatum Anjani	Melastomataceae	Lowering serum glucose;
Momordica charantia Karela / Bittergourd	Cucurbitaceae	Reducing blood glucose level; stimulates glycogen storage by the liver and improves peripheral glucose uptake
Momordica cymbalania, Kadavanchi .	Cucurbitaceae	Reducing blood glucose level ; powdered fruit exhibited hypoglycemic and hypolipidemic properties
Morinda citrifolia Indian Mulberry	Rubiaceae	Aqueous fruit extract decreses Glucose in STZ mice
Morus alba (L.) Shehtut I	Moraceae	Hypoglycemic
Morus indica	Moraceae	Increasing glucose uptake
Mucuna pruriens Kavach / Cowitch	Leguminosae	Reducing blood glucose level
Murraya koeingii Meethi Neem	Rutaceae	Increasing glycogenesis , decrease ;glycogenolysis and gluconeogenesis; aqueous leaves extract shown antihyperglycemic, Hypoglycemic and hypolipidemic effect
Musa sapientum	Musaceae	Reducing blood glucose and glycosylated Hb
Myrtus communis	Myrtaceae	Lowering blood glucose level
Nelumbo nucifera Gaertn. Kamal / Lotus .	Nymphaeaceae	Ethanol extract of its rhizome have antihyperglycemic activity
Nigella sativa (L.) Black	Ranunculaceae	improved glucose tolerance as efficiently as

REVIEW OF LITERATURE

cumin		metformin.
Ocimum gratissimum L.	Lamiaceae	Hypoglycemic
Ocimum sanctum, Tulsi / Basil	Labiatae	Lowering blood sugar level; alcohol extract of its leaves has hypoglycemic effect
Olea europia	Oleaceae	released insulin
Origanum vulgare L.	Lamiaceae	Anti-hyperglycemic activity
Otholobium pubescens (Poir.)	Papilionaceae	Hypoglycemic effect
Paeonia lactiflora Pall.	Paeoniaceae	Blood sugar lowering effect
Pandanus odorus	Pandanaceae	Decreasing plasma glucose level; increases serum insulin levels
Panax ginseng Ginseng	Araliaceae	Lowering blood sugar level antihyperglycemic activity
Parmentieru edulis	Bignoniaceae	Hypoglycemic activity
Picrorrhiza kurroa Kutki.	Scrophulariaceae	potent hypoglycemic activity and delaying of diabetic complications
Piper betle,pan	Piperaceae	Hypoglycemic activity
Plantago ovata Forssk	Plantaginaceae	Antidiabetic activity
Polygala elongata Klein	Polygalaceae	Reduce blood glucose level
Pongamia pinnata (L.) Pierre	Fabaceae	Antidiabetic activity
Psacalium decompositum (A.Gray) H.Rob. & Brettell	Asteraceae	Hypoglycemic activity
Psacalium peltatum (Kunth)	Asteraceae	Anti-hyperglycemic activity
Psidium guajava L.	Myrtaceae	methanol extract showed hypoglycemic effect, ethanol extract showed a marked hypoglycemic

REVIEW OF LITERATURE

		effect
Picrorrhiza kurroa Kalajira	Scrophulariaceae	Its alcohol extract decreasing serum glucose antihyperglycemic, and antilipid-peroxidative effects and enhancement in antioxidants defense system
Phyllanthus amarus Bhui Amla /Indian gooseberry	Euphorbiaceae	Decreasing blood glucose level
Pterocarpus marsupium Roxb. Vijaysar /Indian Malabar .	Fabaceae	Pterostilbene is hypoglycemic in nature
Punica granatum (L.) Anar/ Pomegranate	Punicaceae	Ethanol extract (50%) of its flowers decrese glucose level
Ricinus communis (L.) Eranda/ Gandharva hasta / Castor	Euphorbiaceae	ethanol extract of its roots lower fasting blood glucose
Rosmarinus officinalis (L.)	Labiatae	antihyperglycemic effect and increase serum insulin levels
Retama raetam (Forssk.) Webb	Papilionaceae	Hypoglycemic effect
Salacia oblonga Banaba	Celastraceae	Inhibiting alpha glucosidase activity
Salacia reticulata Kothala himbutu	Celastraceae	Inhibit alpha glucosidase
Sambucus nigra L.	Adoxaceae	Insulin-releasing and insulin-like activity
Sanguis draxonis	Apocynaceae	Increase insulin sensitivity
Sclerocarya birrea (A.Rich.)	Anacardiaceae	Hypoglycemic activity
Scoparia dulcis	Scrophulariaceae	Insulin-secretagogue activity

REVIEW OF LITERATURE

Sweet Broomweed		
Senna occidentalis (L.) Link	Caeslpinaceae	Hypoglycemic activity
Senna sophera (L.) Roxb	Caeslpinaceae	Anti diabetic activity
Senna tora (L.) Roxb.	Caeslpinaceae	Anti diabetic activity
Sida cordifolia (L.) Bala .	*Malvaceae*	The methanol extract have hypoglycemic activity
Solaria oblonga	Celastraceae	Hypoglycemic and possess anti-oxidant activity
Spergularia purpurea (Pers.) G. Don	Caryophyllaceae	Hypoglycemic effect
Suaeda fruticosa	Chenopodiaceae	Hypoglycemic effect
Stevia rebaudiana Bertoni Cheeni Tulsi,	*Asteracea*	Reduces hepatic gluconeogenesis; stimulated insulin
Swertia chirayata Bhuchiretta	Gentianaceae	Stimulating insulin release from islets
Tamarindus indica L. , Tatul tree	Caesalpinaceae	Antidiabetic activity
Telfairia occidentalis Hook.f.	Cucurbitaceae]	Hypoglycemic activity
Terminalia arjuna (Roxb. Ex DC.) Wight & Arn.	Combretaceae	Antidiabetic activity
Terminalia bellirica(Gaertn.)	Combretaceae	Stimulates insulin secretion
Terminalia catappa (L.) Badam/Indian almond.	*Combretaceae*	antihyperglycemic activities in alloxan-induced hyperglycemic rats; β-cells regeneration
Terminalia chebula Retz., Chebulic myrobalan	Combretaceae	Antidiabetic, increases insulin releasefrom the pancreatic islets

REVIEW OF LITERATURE

Terminalia pallida Brandis White Gali nut	*Combretaceae*	ethanol fraction of its fruits showed antihyperglycemic action
Teucrium polium L. Lamiaceae	Lamiaceae	Increases insulin release, antioxidant and hypoglycemic
Tinospora cardifolia Giloe	Menispermaceae	Decreasing blood glucose and brain lipid; showed significant antihyperglycemic activity
Tinospora crispa	Menispermaceae	Anti-hyperglycemic, stimulates insulin release from islets
Trigonella foenum Graceum /Methi	Leguminosae, *Fabaceae*	Decreasing blood glucose concentration; reduce postprandial blood glucose
Triticum repens N'jm L'bouri	Graminae	stimulating glucose uptake by peripheral tissues, inhibiti endogenous glucose production
Urtifca dioica Nettles,	Urticaceae	Increasing insulin secretion
Urtica pilulifera L.	Urticaceae	Hypoglycemic activity
Viburnum opulus Cranberry bush	Caprifoliaceae	Hypoglycemic and Antidiabetic activity
Viscum album	Loranthaceae	Alpha glucosidase inhibitor
Withania coagulans Dunal "Paneer ke phool"	*Solanaceae*	lowered blood sugar and serum cholesterol
Withania somnifera	Solanaceae	Decreasing blood sugar level
Xanthium strumarium	Compositae	Increasing glucose utilization
Zingiber officinale / Adrak/ Ginger	Zingiberaceae	Increasing insulin level and decreasing fasting glucose level
Ziziphus spinachristi Christ thorn	Rhamnaceae	Leaf *n*-butanol fraction and Hydroalcoholic extract have Hypoglycemic activity

2.1.1 Selected plants

On the basis of literature survey, market survey and consulting from traditional drug practitioners *Stevia rebudiana*, *Tinospora cardifolia* and *Triticum aestivum* are selected for study (photograph no.2.1, 2.2 and 2.3).

2.2 *STEVIA REBAUDIANA* (Asteraceae)

Stevia (*Stevia rebudiana Bertoni*) is one of the most efficacious plants, which is an herbaceous perennial plant native to subtropical and tropical rainforest areas of the South America. The basic building block that gives sweet taste to the leaves of the stevia are glycosides was isolated by two French Chemist in 1931.

Bertoni-a French scientist was the first European to document Stevia in 1931 who extracted stevioside from it in the form of an intensely sweet, white crystalline compound. Following this the herb was considered for use as a sweetener during the sugar shortage experienced by Britain during World War II. Since this time, stevia has been used extensively in many Asian and South American countries, but the USA, Canada, Australia and Europe have not embraced the herb as a sweetener, opting either for sugar from readily available sugar-cane or sugar-beet, or for aspartame-based and other artificial sweeteners as a sugar substitute. More than 150 varieties of stevia exist, but *S. rebaudiana* Bertoni is the only sweet stevia species. Carbohydrate-based compounds from the stevia leaf can be isolated to glycosides which are glycosides of the diterpene derivative steviol, and is a natural component of the plant. Stevioside is intensely sweet and is present up to 13 % in its leaves. Rebaudiosides and dulcosides are other sweet constituents of the plant found in lesser quantity.

REVIEW OF LITERATURE

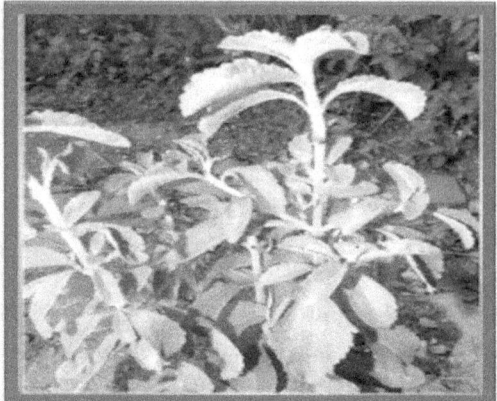

Photograph 2.1 *Stevia rebudiana*

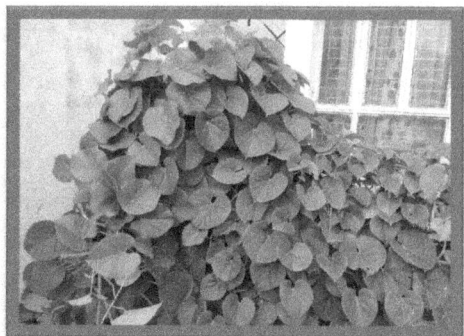

Photograph 2.2 *Tinospora cardifolia*

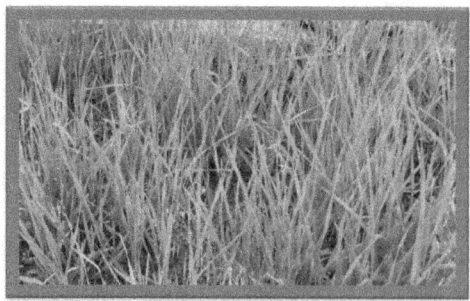

Photograph 2.3 *Triticum aestivum*

REVIEW OF LITERATURE

2.2.1 Scientific Classification

Kingdom	Plantae
Division	Magnoliophyta
Class	Magnoliophyta
Order	Asteraces
Family	Asteraceae
Genus	*Stevia*
Species	*rebaudiana*

2.2.2 Vernacular Names

Hindi	Cheeni tulsi
Marathi	Madhu parani
Punjabi	Gurmar
Sanskrit	Madhu patra
Tamil	Seeni tulsi
Telgu	Madhu patri

2.2.3 Plant Description

S. rebaudiana - a member of family Asteraceae is a native of Paraguay where it grows in sandy soils near streams **(Katayama *et al.*, 1976)**. The well-drained red soil and sandy loam soil should have the pH range of 6.5- 7.5. Saline soil should be avoided to cultivate this plant. It is a small shrubby perennial growing up to 65 cm tall, with sessile, oppositely arranged lanceolate to oblanceolate leaves, serrated above the middle, about 5 cm long and 2 cm wide and facing each other. The flowers are small (7-15 mm), white and arranged in an irregular cyme. The seed is an achene with a feathery pappus. The plants can be used for commercial production for 6 years, during which it can be harvested five times a year above the ground **(Robinson, 1930)**.

2.2.4 Phytochemical profile

In 1931 two French chemists, Bridel and Lavieille, isolated diterpene glycosides from leaves of *S. rebaudiana*. In **Cramer and Ikan 1987,** reported basic structure of diterpene glycoside and stated order of various sweet associated derivative glycosides **(Table 2.2)**. Moreover stevia leaves contain a complex mixture of natural diterpene glycosides namely, steviol, steviolbioside, stevioside, rebaudioside A-F and ducloside A, which are responsible for the typical sweet taste **(Figure 2.1) (Mantovaneli *et al.*, 2004)**. Apart from that, **McGarvey *et al.*, (2003)** reported non-sweet secondary compounds as labdane diterpene, triterpenes, sterols, flavonoids, volatile oil constituents, pigments, gums and inorganic matter and other chemicals such as Apigenin-4'-o-beta-d-glucoside, austroinulin, avicularin, beta-sitosterol, caffeic acid, campesterol, caryophyllene, centaureidin, chlorogenic acid, chlorophyll, cosmosiin, cynaroside, daucosterol, diterpene glycosides, dulcosides A-B, foeniculin, formic acid, gibberellic acid, gibberellin, indole-3-acetonitrile, isoquercitrin, isosteviol, jhanol, kaempferol-3-o-rhamnoside, kaurene, lupeol, luteolin-7-o-glucoside, polystachoside, quercetin, quercitrin, scopoletin, sterebin A-H, steviolmonoside, stigmasterol, umbelliferone and xanthophylls.

According to Sharma et al. (2006), the fresh Stevia leaves contain a large amount of water between 80 and 85%. The main constituents present were glycosides such as stevioside, steviol and rebaudioside A and B. The other constituents present in Stevia were ascorbic acid, b-carotene, chromium, cobalt, magnesium, iron, potassium, phosphorous, riboflavin, thiamin, tin, zinc, and so forth. The other chemicals found in Stevia include apigenin, austroinulin, avicularin, b-sitosterol, caffeic acid, compesterol, caryophyllene, centaureidin, chorogenic acid, chlorophyll, cynaroside, daucosterol, di-terpene glycoside, dulcosides A and B, foeniculin, formic acid, gibberellic acid, gibberellin, indole-3-acetonitrile, isoquercitrin, isosteviol, kaempferol, kaurene,

lupeol, luteolin, polysatachoside, quercetin, quercitrin, scooletin, stigmasterol, umbelliferone and xanthophyllus. The leaves of *Stevia* contain a natural complex mixture of eight sweet diterpene glycosides, including isosteviol, stevioside, rebaudiosides (A, B, C, D, E, F), steviolbio-side and dulcoside A **(Goyal et al., 2010)**. Out of various steviol glycosides (SGs), stevioside and rebaudioside A are the major metabolites and these compounds are 250 to 300 times as sweet as sucrose **(Allam et al., 2001; Mantovaneli et al., 2004;)**, pH-stable, heat-stable, not fermentable.

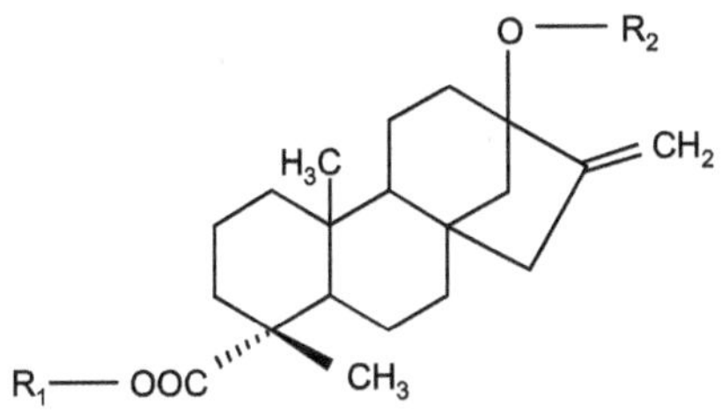

Figure 2.1 : Basic structure of diterpene glycosides of *S. rebaudiana*

REVIEW OF LITERATURE

Table 2.2 : Classification of sweet diterpene glycosides of *S. rebaudiana*

Diterpene glycoside	R_1^a	R_2^a
Steviolbioside	H	$glc^2\text{—}^1glc$
Rubusoside	glc	Glc
Stevioside	glc	$glc^2\text{—}^1glc$
Rebaudioside A	glc	$glc_3^2\text{—}^1glc$ $\searrow ^1glc$
Rebaudioside B	H	$glc_3^2\text{—}^1glc$ $\searrow ^1glc$
Rebaudioside C (dulcoside B)	glc	$glc_3^2\text{—}^1rhm$ $\searrow ^1glc$
Rebaudioside D	$glc^2\text{—}^1glc$	$glc_3^2\text{—}^1glc$ $\searrow ^1glc$
Rebaudioside E	$glc^2\text{—}^1glc$	$glc^2\text{—}^1glc$
Dulcoside B	glc	$glc^2\text{—}^1rham$

[a]glc, β-D-glucopyranosyl; rham, α-L-rhamnopyranosyl

2.2.5 Pharmacological Activities

○ **Antidiabetic activities:**

Stevia leaves have a significant role in alleviating damage in the streptozotocin-diabetic rats besides its hypoglycemic effect and it also reduce the risk of oxidative stress **(Shivanna et al., 2013)**.

Chen et al 2005, suggested that leaf extract of *S. rebaudiana* (200 and 400 mg/kg) significantly reduce blood glucose level, without producing condition of hypoglycemia after treatment, together with lesser loss in the body weight as compared with standard positive control drug glibenclamide

As per **Gregersen et al., 2004** stevioside is beneficial for treatment of Type-2 diabetes. **Jeppesen et al., 2000** documented stevioside and steviol as potent antihyperglycemic agents.

Stevia also has been used to control weight in obese persons and it may be presumed that it is advantageous for obesity laden diabetes **(Suttajit et al., 1993)**.

Curi et al., 1986, showed that treatment with *S. rebaudiana* increases glucose tolerance.

Misra et al., 2011 showed that it decrease plasma glucose concentrations.

As per **Yang et al., 2010,** Stevioside has the ability to activate peripheral μ-opoid receptor for lowering plasma glucose and to increase glycogen synthesis in liver.

Maki et al., 2008, concluded chronic consumption of 1000 mg of rebaudioside A, a steviol glycoside in men and women with Type-2 diabetes does not alter glucose homeostasis or blood pressure.

Ferreira et al., 2006 decreases glucose concentration in fasted rats, which may occur by reduction of hepatic gluconeogenesis, inhibition of pyruvate carboxylase and phosphoenol PEPCK pathway.

Chen et al.,2006, reported that stevioside counteracts the glyburide-induced desensitization of the pancreatic β-cells function in mice.

Chen et al., 2005, showed stevioside improve insulin level in diabetic rats.

Suanarunsawat et al., 2004 reported suppression of glucagons are the primary cause of antihyperglycemic effect of stevioside in diabetic mice.

Abudula et al., 2004, concluded Rebaudioside-A, potentially stimulates insulin secretion from isolated mouse islets and possesses insulinotropic effect and therefore may serve a potential role in treatment of Type-2 diabetes mellitus.

REVIEW OF LITERATURE

○ **Cardiovascular activity:**

Barriocanal *et al.*, 2008, concluded that consumption of steviol glycosides in humans as a sweetener by normal and diabetic subjects, including those with normal / low-normal blood pressure is safe and dose not produce hypoglycemia or hypotension.

Ferri *et al.*, 2006 studied that crude stevioside up to 15.0 mg/kg/day did not show an antihypertensive effect.

As per **Hsieh *et al.*, 2003,** Previous animal and human studies have indicated that stevioside has an antihypertensive effect.

Hseih *et al.*, 2003 observed significant alleviation in BP compared to placebo control groups.

Hsu *et al.*, 2002, found that stevioside given at the concentration of 100,200 and 400 mg/kg i.p. lowered blood pressure dose dependently in spontaneously hypertensive rats (SHR).

Lee *et al.*, 2001, study has shown that intra peritoneal injection of stevioside at dose of 25mg/kg has antihypertensive effect in spontaneously hypertensive rats.

Chan *et al.*, 2000 suggested that oral stevioside is a well tolerated and effective modality which may be considered as an alternative or supplementary therapy for hypertensive patients.

Immunological potential:

Takasaki *et al.*, (2009) study suggested that stevioside, as well as steviol and isosteviol, could be valuable as chemo-preventive agents for chemical carcinogenesis.

Sehar *et al.*, (2008) result revealed that stevioside is found effective in increasing phagocytic activity, haemagglutination antibody titre and delayed type hypersensitivity. Therefore drug hold promise as an immunomodulating agent by stimulating both humoral as well as cellular immunity.

Boonkaewwan et al., (2006) proposed that stevioside attenuates synthesis of inflammatory mediators in lipo-polysaccharide (LPS) stimulated THP-1 cells by interfering with the IKK beta and NF-Kappa B signaling pathway, and stevioside-induced TNF-α secretion is partially mediated through TLR4.

Yasukawa et al., (2002) revealed inhibitory effect of stevioside on tumor promotion by 12-o-tetradecanoyl phorbol-13-acetate in two-stage carcinogenesis in mouse skin.

- **Antidiuretic activity:**

    Melis et al., (1999) screened the anti-diuretic activity of crude extract of *S. rebaudiana* leaves in male wister rats where result has shown that extract significantly increased reabsorption of water by collecting duct and exert water diuresis by increasing of free water clearance.

- **Gastrointestinal functions:**

    In Brazil, stevia is used to flavor the bitter medicinal preparations, to improve digestion and overall gestrointestinal function. Likewise in China, stevia is used as a low calorie, sweet tasting tea, as an appetite stimulant, as a digestive aid and as an aid to losing weight and even for staying young **(Ray, 2008)**.

- **Antimicrobial activity:**

    Manish et al., (2006) studied antimicrobial activity of various extract of *S. rebaudiana* leaves. Where water extract have shown activity against *B. subtilis* and *S. aureus*, methanol extract gave the highest zone of inhibition against *P. aeruginosa*.

    According to **Tomita et al., (1997)** fermented hot water extracts of *S. rebaudiana* have shown significant bactericidal activities for enterohemorrhagic *Escherichia coli* O157: H7 and other food-borne pathogenic bacteria in acidic condition.

- **Antifertility activity:**

    As per **Melis et al., (1999)** *S. rebaudiana* decreases the plasma testosterone level, and may decrease the fertility of male rats.

REVIEW OF LITERATURE

Yodyingyuad *et al.*, (1991) studied that daily fed stevioside at dose of 0.5. 1.0 and 2.5-g/kg bw/day respectively showed that no abnormality found in growth in fertility in both sexes.

Oliveira-Filho *et al.*, (1989) suggested that in male rat's seminal vesicle weight was found to be reduced which presumed that chronic consumption of *S. rebaudiana* leave extract has crippling fertility while endocrine system may have some influence over this activity.

Miscellaneous activity:

According to **Xu *et al.*, (2008)** the neuroprotective effect of isosteviol against cerebral ischemia injury induced by middle cerebral artery occlusion in rats.

Hong *et al.*, (2006) reported that stevioside reduces the release of glucagon. According to **Wong *et al.*, (2006)** isosteviol (a metabolite of steviol) inhibits angiotention-11-induced cell proliferation and endothelin-1-secretion both of which have been implicated in the pathogenesis of chronic vascular diseases.

2.2.6 Safety Issues

Stevioside and rebaudioside-A are not genotoxic *in-vivo* or *in-vitro*. **(Benford *et al.*, 2009)**. Phytoconstituents of *S.rebaudiana*, including steviol, stevioside and rebaudiosides etc., are likely to be safe when used as a sweetener in foods. Following precautions during pregnancy and in other disease conditions should be kept in mind.

Pregnancy and breast-feeding:

Not enough and satisfactory data yet had been established about the use of

S. rebaudiana during pregnancy and breast-feeding.

Low blood pressure:

There is some evidence, though not conclusive, that some of the constituents of *S. rebaudiana* can lower blood pressure and there is a concern that its phytoconstituents might have caused blood pressure to drop too low in people who have low blood pressure.

REVIEW OF LITERATURE

2.3. *TINOSPORA CORDIFOLIA*

Tinospora cordifolia is an important drug of Indian systems of medicine and used in medicines since times immemorial. It belongs to family Menispermaceae. It is a glabrous, succulent, woody climbing shrub native to India. It is also found in Burma and Sri Lanka. In Hindi, the plant is commonly known as Giloya, Giloe or Amrita. Giloya is a Hindu mythological term that refers to the heavenly elixir which has saved celestial beings from old age and kept them eternally young. Guduchi, the Sanskrit name means one which protects the entire body. The term 'Amrita' is attributed to its ability to impart youthfulness and longevity (**Raghu et al., 2006; Wealth of India 1966, Nadkarni 1976**).

2.3.1 Taxonomic Classification

Kingdom	-	Plantae
Division	-	Magnoliophyta
Class	-	Magnoliopsida
Order	-	Ranunculales
Family	-	Menispermaceae
Geneus	-	*Tinospora*
Species	-	*cordifolia*

2.3.2 Vernacular Names

Hindi	–	Kareli
Bengali	–	Karala, Kerula, Uchchhe
Hindi	–	Giloe
Bengali	–	Gulancha
Kannada	–	Amrtaballi
Malayalam	–	Amrtu
Tamil	–	Amarutavalli
Telugu	–	Amrta
Marathi	–	Gulvel
Oriya	–	Theisawntlung
Gujarathi	-	Galo

2.3.3 Botanical Description :

The bark of *T. cordifolia* is creamy white to grey, deeply left spirally, the space in between being spotted with large rosette like lenticels. The wood is white, soft and porous and the fleshy cut surface quickly assumes a yellow tint on exposure to air. The branches bear smooth heart-shaped leaves, unisexual greenish flowers and red berries. The male flowers are clustered and female are usually solitary. The leaves are simple, alternate with long petiole and possess a characteristic heart shape, giving the name cordifolia to the plant. The drupes are ovoid, glossy, succulent, red and pea-sized (**Photograph 2**). The seeds are curved. Fruits are fleshy and single seeded. Flowers grow during the summer and fruits during the winter. The odour is not characteristic, but the taste is bitter **(Wealth of India 1966)**.

2.3.4 Phytochemical Profile of *T. cordifolia* :

A large number of compounds belonging to different classes such as alkaloids, diterpenoid lactones, steroids, glycosides aliphatic compounds, polysaccharides. Some constituents have been isolated from plant mainly they are tinosporone, tinosporic acid, cordifolisides A to E, syringen, berberine, giloin, gilenin, crude giloininand, arabinogalactan polysaccharide, picrotene, bergenin, gilosterol, tinosporol, tinosporidine, sitosterol, cordifol, heptacosanol, octacosonal, tinosporide, columbin, chasmanthin, palmarin, palmatosides C and F, amritosides, cordioside, tinosponone, ecdysterone, makisterone A, hydroxyecdysone, magnoflorine, tembetarine, syringine, glucan polysaccharide, syringine apiosylglycoside, isocolumbin, palmatine, tetrahydropalmaitine, jatrorrhizine aliphatic compounds and polysaccharides are present *T.cordifolia*. Its leaves are rich in protein (11.2%), calcium and phosphorus.(**SS Singh et al.,2003**)(Fig 2.2)

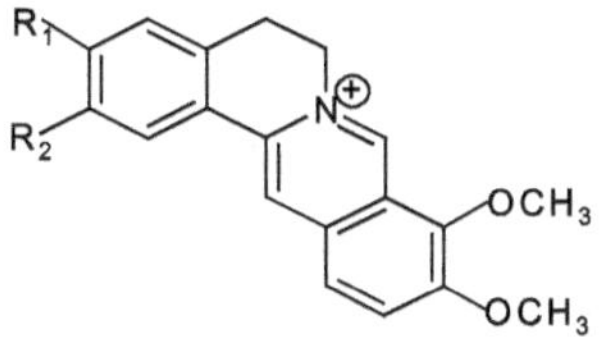

(i) $R_1, R_2 = O - CH_2 - O$
(ii) $R_1 = R_2 = OCH_3$

(i) Berberine (ii) Palmatine

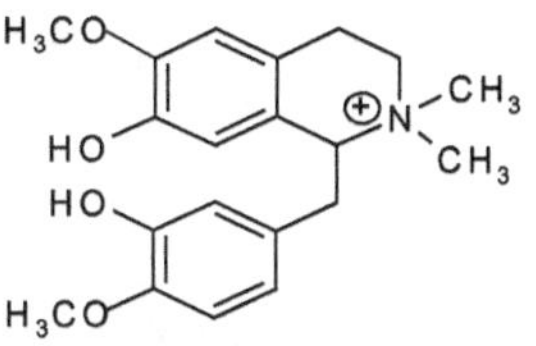

(iii) **Magnoflorine**

Fig. 2.2: Some bioactive compounds from *T.cordifolia*

REVIEW OF LITERATURE

Table 2.3: Phytoconstituents of *T.cordifolia* with their bio-spectrum

Type of chemical	Active principle	Part
Alkaloid	Berberine, Palmatine, Tembetarine, Magnoflorine, Choline, Tinosporin, Isocolumbin, Tetrahydropalmatine, Aporphinealkaloids, Jatrorrhizine, Tetrahydropalmatine	Stem and root
Glycosides	18-norclerodane glucoside, furanoid diterpene glucoside, Tinocordiside, Tinocordifolioside, Syringin, Palmatosides, Cordifoliside A-E, 18-norclerodane, glucoside, Cordioside, Syringinapiosylglycoside, Pregnane glycoside, Palmatosides	Stem
Diterpenoid lactone	Furanolactone, tinosporon, tinosporides, Jateorine, columbin, clerodane derivatives, Furanolactone, Clerodane derivatives, [(5R,10R)-4R-8Rdihydroxy-2S-3R:15,16-diepoxy-clerroda-13 (16),14-dieno-17,12S:18,1Sdilactone],Tinosporon, Tinosporides, Jateorine, Columbin	Whole plant
Steroid	β-sitosterol, δ-sitosterol, 20 β-hydroxy ecdysone, ecdysterone, makisterone A, giloinsterol	Aerial part stem
Sesquiterpenoid	Tinocordifolin	Stem
Aliphatic compound	Octacosanol, Heptacosanol, Nonacosan-15-one	Whole plant
Miscellaneous compound	Jatrorrhizine, cordifol, tinoporidine, cordifeline, giloin, giloinin, Tinosporic acid	Whole plant

2.3.5 Pharmacological Activity : *T. cordifolia* has following pharmacological activities:-

(a)　Immunomodulating activity:

Upadhyay PR et al 2011, suggested that *T. cordifolia* strength the immune system in a variety of ways. Syringin, cordioside and cordifolioside were found to possess immunopotentiating activity.

As per **Kalikar *et al.*, (2008)** *T. cordifolia* extract (TCE), significantly affected the symptoms of HIV. TCE treatment caused significant reduction in eosinophil count and hemoglobin percentage. 60% patients receving TCE and 20% on placebo reported decrease in the incidence of various symptoms associated with disease.

As per **Nair *et al.*, 2004** Alpha-D-glucan separated from *T. cordifolia* exhibits immunoprotective and immunostimulatory effect.

According to **Manjrekar *et al.*, (2000)**, water and ethanol extracts of stems of *T. cordifolia* and *T. sinensis* inhibit immunosuppression produced by Cyclophosphamide. Ethanol extracts of stems of these plants inhibit cyclophosphamide-induced anemia.

According to **Chintelwar *et al.*, 1999** An arabinogalactan isolated from the dired stems of *T. cordifolia* and examined by methylation analysis, partial hydrolysis and carboxyl reduction, has shown polyclonal mitogenic activity against B-cell, their proliferation did not require macrophage.

As per **Kapil and Sharma, 1997** the active principles of *T. cordifolia* have anticomplementary and immunomodulatory activities. It increase in IgG antibodies in serum. Humoral and cell mediated immunity were also enhanced depending upon the given dose.

Atal *et al.*, 1986 reported that administration of an aqueous suspension of a 95% ethanol stem extract of *T.cordifolia* to mice (100mg/kg,p.o) increased phagocytic activity of the reticuloendothelial system without affecting the humoral or cell-mediated immunity.

(b) Anti-Cancer Activity

Bala et al, 2015, studied anticancer activity of secondary metabolites from *Tinospora cordifolia* against four different human cancer cell lines, KB (human oral squamous carcinoma), CHOK-1(hamster ovary), HT-29 (human colon cancer) and SiHa (human cervical cancer) and murine primary cells respectively. All extracts and fractions were active against KB and CHOK-1 cells whereas among the pure molecules palmatine was found to be active against KB and HT-29; tinocordiside against KB and CHOK-1;yangambin against KB cells.

Puttananjaiah et al, 2015 reported that hexane and methanol fractions of *Tinospora cordifolia* suppressed the proliferation, migration and invasion of MCF-7cells.

Tinospora cordifolia shows anti-cancer activity. According to **Ali and Dixit , 2013,** alkaloid palmatine from *Tinospora cordifolia* indicate the anticancer potential in 7,12-dimethylbenz(a)anthracene DMBA induced skin cancer model in mice.

Mishra and Kaur,2013, suggested the anti-brain cancer potential of 50% ethanolic extract of *Tinospora cordifolia* (TCE) using C6 glioma cells.

Verma R. et al;2011, reported that 50% methanolic extract of *Tinospora cordifolia* at a dose 750 mg/kg body weight for 30 days showed increase in life span and tumor size was significantly reduced as compared to control in C57 Bl mice when received.

According to **Singh et al., (2006)** TC is potent chemopreventive agent against various diseases including cancer as it induces enzymes of carcinogen/drug metabolism and antioxidant system. alcoholic extract of *T. cordifolia* influence the myeloid differentiation of bone marrow progenitor cells and the recuitment of macrophages in response to tumor growth *in situ*.

Jagetia and Rao, (2006) observed, antitumor, properties of dichloromethane extract of Guduchi and reported that cytotoxic effect of this extract may be due to lipid peroxidation and release of LDH and decline in GST. They

Jagetia et al., (2005) suggested that cytotoxic effects of methylene chloride (dichloromethane) stem extract of *T. cordifolia* could be due to DNA damage, inhibition of topoisomerase II, increased lipid peroxidation (TBARS) and lactate dehydrogenase (LDH) accompanied by a decrease in glutathione-s-transferase.

Singh *et al.*, (2005) observed that *in vivo* administration of alcohol extract of *T. cordifolia* to mice bearing a spontaneous T cell lymphoma designated as Dalton's lymphoma prevented tumor growth dependent regression of thymus. It restored thymus homeostasis and increases survival of tumor bearing mice.

Levon and Kuttan, 2004 concluded that intraperitoneal administration of the polysaccharide fraction of *T. cordifolia* (stem) at dose of 0.5 mg to C57BL/6 mice for 10 days simultaneously with the injection BI6F10 melanoma cells significantly inhibited (72%) metastases formation, increased survival time (>2-fold) and significantly reduced biochemical markers (hydroxyproline, hexosamines" uronic acids, and serum y-glutamyl-transpeptidase and sialic acid levels) of metastases.

Jagetia *et al*, 1998, reported that the effect of Giloy is better in respect to doxorubicin treatment.

Dhar *et al.*, 1968 reported 50% ethanol stem extract of *T. cordifolia* exhibiting antitumourigenic activity against sarcoma 180, hepatoma 129 and Friend virus leukaemia in the mouse, but not against other test systems investigated.

(c)   **Anti-diabetic activity:**

Sangeetha et al, 2011, reported that TC stem cure diabetes by regulating level of blood glucose.

As per **Chougale et al, 2009** ethyl acetate, dichloromethane, chloroform and hexane extract of TC stem inhibits the amylase and glucosidase enzymes due to which post-prandial glucose level decreases.

Umamaheswari and Mainzen , 2007 reported root extract of this plant decrease the level of glycosylated haemoglobin and hydroperoxidase.

As per **Grover *et al.*, 2002;** aqueous extract of *T. cordifolia* at 400 mg/day for 50 days show hypoglycemic effect on day 60 in diabetic mice.

REVIEW OF LITERATURE

According to **Grover et al., 2001,** regular use of *T. cordifolia* extract decreases blood glucose level in rodents.

T. cordifolia treatment decreased degree of tissue damage in the diabetic model was evidenced through the improved total haemoglobin levels, body weight gain, increased hepatic hexokinase and reduced hepatic glucose-6-phosphatase**(Prince and Menon, 2000)**.

A constituent ($C_{32}H_{61}NO_3$) from TC stem showed hypoglycemic activity at 0.2 mg/kg in the oral GTT over 3 h for fasted rabbits**(Mahajan and Jolly, 1985 and Grover et al., 2000)**.

Both the organic (250 mg/kg of a dried 95% ethanol extract) and inorganic (90 mg pure ash/kg) components of the *T. cordifolia* stem exhibited hypoglycemic effects in the oral glucose tolerance test over 3 h for fasted Charles Foster Strain white albino rats where the effect of the inorganic components was more pronounced **(Kar et al., 1999)**.

Aqueous, alcohol and chloroform extract of the leaves of *T. cordifolia* showed dose dependent (50, 100, 150 or 200 mg/kg, p.o) hypoglycemic activity rabbits at 50-100 mg/kg **(Wadood et al., 1992)**.

TC aqueous extract (400mg/kg) to male rabbits significantly inhibited adrenaline-induced hyperglycaemia. **(Raghunathan and Sharma, 1969)**.

According to **Dhar et al., (1968)**, a dried 50% ethanol stem extract exerted hypoglycemic activity in fasted albino rats.

(d)   Hypolipidemic activity:

Stanely et al., 1999 studied TC roots aqueous extract restore lipid profile in alloxan diabetic rats.

(e)   Antioxidant effects:

According to **Jayaprakash et al, 2015** in nitrosodiethylamine (DEN) induced liver cancer TC ethanolic extract reverted the lipid peroxidation in male Wister albino rats.

Sharma *et al*; 2012, study results suggested that *Tinospora cordifolia* bark ethanol extracts showed the highest free radical scavenging activity compared to the methanol extracts and also ethanol extracts had the highest phenol content.

As per **Goel and Prem Kumar, (2002)** TC aqueous extract inhibit fenton reaction and radiation mediated degradation.

Prince and Menon, 2000 showed regular use of aqueous root extract decreased plasma thiobarbituric acid reactive substances, ceruloplasmin and α-tocopherol and increased plasma glutathione, vitamin C and superoxide dismutase.

(f)   Hepato-protective activity:

According to **Bishayi, 2002**, *T. cordifolia* extract protect the liver (100 mg/kg body weight for 15 days) in CCl_4 liver toxicity in rats.

Nagarkatli *et al*., 1994 reported kupffer cell function suppressed in liver damage is protected by *T. cordifolia* pretreatment.

As per **Rege *et al*., 1993**, when patients were given *T.cordifolia* extract orally during biliary drainage alongwith vitamin K and antibiotics, it was concluded that *T. cordifolia* improves the drainage by strengthening host defense.

As per **Rege *et al*., 1984**, acute liver damage induced by carbon-tetrachloride was exacerbated by *T. cordifolia* (100mg/kg, p.o) pretreatment, while long term (≤12 weeks) co-administration of *T. cordifolia* (100mg/kg, p.o) with CCl_4 appeared to help prevent fibrous changes and promote regeneration by parenchymal tissues.

(g) Anti-Microbial Activity

Francesca B. et al 2014, concluded that TC constituents inhibit activity of Staphylococcus aureus and Klebsiella pneumoniae.

Singh et al 2014 Silver nanoparticles synthesized from stem of *Tinospora cordifolia* possess very good antibacterial activity against multidrugresistantstrains of Pseudomonas aeruginosa isolated from burn patients.

Shanthi and Nelson 2013 leaves and stem extracts of TC inhibit activity of Klebsiella pneumoniae and Pseudomonas aeruginosa.

Veeramuthu D. et al 2012 showed *Tinospora cordifolia* stem ethanol extract have activity against bacteria and fungi.

(h) Anti-Toxic Activity

Hamsa and Kuttan 2012, indicated that *Tinospora cordifolia* reduced Cyclophosphamide induced toxicities in cancer treatment.

Gupta and Sharma 2011, reported that *Tinospora cordifolia* extracts scavenge free radicals generated during aflatoxicosis.

According to **Shanish et al; 2010,** TC crude powder reduced the toxicity of L-DOPA therapy in Parkinson's disease.

Sharma and Pandey 2010, reported that Leaf and stem extract of T. cordifolia showed hepatoprotective activity in albino mice.

(i)   Antistress activity:

According to **Singh et al., 2003** root of *T. cordifolia* are useful in stress.

Sarma et al., 1997 reported that alcohol root extract of *T. cordifolia* possess some normalising activity against 8h restrain stress, induced changes in brain norepinephrine, dopamine, 5-hydroxy-tryptamine and 5-hydroxyindoleacetic acid levels in Charles-Foster male rats when administered at 100mg/kg/day, p.o for 16 days.

(j)   Anti-inflammatory activity:

According to **Naidu et al., 1990,** *T. cordifolia* reduce the pain and morning sickness associated with rheumatoid arthritis.

Pendse et al., 1977 resulted that *T. cordifolia* was effective in acute inflammation. But in subacute inflammation.

REVIEW OF LITERATURE

As per **Shah and Pandhya, 1976,** in formalin induced arthritis TC showed anti-inflammatory effect.

(k) Artipyretic activity:

According to **Spelman, 2001** traditionally TC used in fever.

Vedavathy and Rao, 1991 concluded that water soluble fractions of a 95% ethanol extract of whole *T. cordifolia* showed significant antipyretic activity in albino rats which were given 500 mg/kg, p.o following yeast-induced pyrexia.

As per **Lehari *et al.*, 1984,** its aqueous stem extract showed slight but insignificant antipyretic effect in rabbits following yeast-induced pyrexia.

(l) Anti-infective and antiallergic activity:

Jeyachandran *et al.*, 2003, showed that ethanol extract of TC stem have antibacterial activity against *E. coli, Proteus valgaris, Enterobacter faecalis, Salmonella typhi (gram –ve), Staphylococcus aureus* and *Serratia marcescens*, while chloroform extract of stem showed moderate inhibition to 4 of the test organisms excluding *Staphylococcus aureus* and *Serratia marcescens* while aqueous extract displayed slight antibacterial activity against *E. coli*] **Spelman, 2001** reported aqueous extract of *T. cordifolia* reduces bronchospasm in guinea pigs.

Sharma *et al.*, 1990, reported TC extract in cure patients suffering from urticaria.

(m) Radioprotective effects:

According to **Goel *et al.*, 2004** administration of a 50% alcoholic stem extract of *T. cordifolia* (200 mg/kg, i.p) showed radioprotective activity when given before .gamma-irradiation.

Subramanian *et al.*, 2003, reported that the entire radioprotective activity of a polysaccharide preparation of *T cordifolia* can be attributed to its radical scavenging capacity.

REVIEW OF LITERATURE

(n) **Miscellaneous experimental studies:**

Rao et al., 2005 cocluded that *T. cordifolia* alcoholic extract in a rat model in surgically induced myocardial ischemia where they observed that it is pretreatment cardioprotective and limits ischemia reperfusion induced myocardial infraction.

Badar et al., 2005 reported that TC extracts decreased symptoms of allergic rhinitis in patients.

2.4 *Triticum aestivum*

Wheatgrass have numerous therapeutic and nutritional properties. TA is rich in nutritious supplements.

2.4.1 Taxonomical Classification

Kingdom	-	Plantae
Division	-	Magnoliophyta
Class	-	Liliopsida
Order	-	Cyperales
Family	-	Poaceae
Geneus	-	*Triticum* L.
Species	-	*Triticum aestivum*

2.4.2 Vernacular Names

Hindi: Gehun

Kannada: Godhi

Manipuri: Gehun

Marathi: Gehun

Sanskrit: bahudugdha

Tamil: godumbaiyarisi

Telugu: godumalu

2.4.3 Botanical Description

Young leaves of wheat plants are known as Wheatgrass (TA). It's culms are simple and pithy. The leaves are flat and narrow, spikes are long and dorsally compressed.

2.4.4 Phytochemical profile

The major chemical constituents WG are amino acids, vitamins, Chlorophyll, enzyme, bioflavonoid and indole compounds. Among amino acids, leucine, iso leucien, threonine, valine, threonine, phenylalanine, tryptophane, metheonine etc are found in TA. vitamin A, B-complex, E, C and K are present in high quantity. Iron, calcium, phosphorus, megnasium, zinc, copper, sodium, sulfur, boron, molybdenum and iodine forms it's major part. Protease, amylase, lipase, cytochrome oxidase, trans hydrogenase, superoxide dismutase and malic dehydrogenase enzymes are present in it. Apigenin, quercitin, luteonin are, choline and amygdalin are also present in wheat grass. **(Singh, N. 2005; Meyerowitz S. 1992; Rajesh and Ramesh,2011)**

2.4.5 Pharmacological Activity :

(a) Anticancer activity:

Padalia *et al* ., 2010 and Ben – Arye ., 2002, proved that wheat grass detoxify the body.

Mukopadhyay *et al.*, 2009, showed by clinical studies that in myelodysplastic syndrome WG reduce serum ferritin.

Pratt *et al.*, 1992 and Egner *et al.*, 2001 reported in cancer it provide beneficial effect.

Bar – Sela *et al* , 2007, reported that WG contains enzymes that help to protect us from carcinogens, including superoxides dismutase (SOD) that lesser the effect of radiations.

Dey *et al.*, 2006 found that in cancer patients it improve the health status.

Marwah *et al.*, 2004, evaluated that in Beta- Thalassemia it give beneficial effect on the transfusion requirement.

Padalia *et al* ., 2010 and Ben – Arye *et al* ., 2002, proved that wheat grass helps in blood flow, digestion and detoxification of the body

As per Falcioni *et al* ., 2002, Wheat grass helps to neutralize toxins and environmental pollutants in the body.

According to Christne *et al* ., 2001, it's indole compounds increasing the activity of xenobiotic metabolic due to which carcinogens are deactivated.

According to Andrew et al 2000, Hemila H. 1992 and Chernomorsky and Segelman 1988 Chlorophyll inhibits the metabolic activity of carcinogens.

(b) Anti- Ulcer Activity

As per Shah , 2007, bioflavonoid, api- genin, inhibit tumour necrosis factor (TNF) induced transactivation.

According to **Singha and, Prince, 2004; WG** rich in bioflavonoid so it is useful in ulcerative colitis

According to **Ben-Arye *et al.*, 2002** it is useful in Ulcerative colitis.

Chernomorsky and Segelman,1988 suggested that it acts as wound healing agent.

(c) Blood Related Diseases

According to **Fibach *et al.*, 1993; Fernandes and O'Donovan, 2005; Reynolds C 2005;** WG is useful in anaemia, high blood pressure, atherosclerosis and internal haemorrhage.

Soma *et al.*,2008 showed beneficial effects of WG supplementation in patients having hemolytic disorders.

(d) Antidiabetic activity:

According to **Rana *et al;* 2011** WG improve digestive system problems especially in Diabetes.

(e) Anti- Oxidant Activity

According to **Aydos *et al*., 2011** wheat grass increase activity of CAT and SOD.

Tandon *et al.*, 2011 studied that MCF-7 breast cancer lines with different extracts show highest free radical scavenging activity.

Kulkarni *et al.*, 2006 and Siener *et al*, 2006 determined that it has lipid per oxidation activity.

(f) Anti- Arthritic Activity : .

Mujoriya R,2011 and **Rana *et al;* 2011** reported Anti- Arthritic Activity of WG.

Nenonen *et al* ., 1998; observed positive effect of WG in arthritic patients

(g) Anti-asthmatic and Anti-allergic agent

REVIEW OF LITERATURE

According to **Prasad AS, 2008,** its constituent Zn and Mg reduces inflammatory cytokines and produce bronchodilatation.

Kamat et al., 2000, reported that luteolin and quercitin interfere with secretion of histamine, leukotrienes and prostaglandin.

(h) Digestive diseases:

Wheat grass therapy is useful in digestive disorders. It act as laxative in rectal bleeding and chronic constipation.

(i) General cure

According to **Sean M, 2002** wheatgrass is good for general weakness, insomnia, headache, fever, etc..

Bar-Sela et al., 2007 and Dey S et al., 2006 showed that it removes toxins and clean the blood.

(j) Promotes healthy skin:

According to **Ben-Arye et al.,2002, Christne et al.,2001, Shah S 2007** WG give young look, and restore the signs of aging.

2.4.6 Safety Issues:

It should be avoided to those person who are hypersensitive to any component of TA.

Pregnancy and Breastfeeding

As per **Sean M, 2002,** TA may be contaminated with microbs so raw TAs not recommended for pregnant or breastfeeding women.

Adverse reactions:

Nausea and headache occurs due to excess quantity. Hypersensitive person may suffer from swelling of throat. Persons those taking warfarin should avoid TA because it contains higher concentration of vitamin K.

PHARMACOGNOSTIC STUDY

3.1 Identification of Collected Plant Materials

Stevia rebaudiana leaves and *Tinospora cordifolia* leaves and stems authentified by the Botany Department Saifia Science college Bhopal (M.P), after collecting from the areas in and around Bhopal. Voucher specimens were deposited (420/ Bot./saf./14 and421/ Bot./saf./14). For cultivation of *Triticum aesitivum*, sensible quality wheat cleansed, soaked in water then tied in wet cotton cloth for germination. Germinated wheat was sowed in soil. On the 9th day, the grass reached the length of 16 to 18cm which was then Collected and authenticated by the Botany Department Saifia Science college, Bhopal (M.P) and voucher specimens were deposited (422/ Bot./saf./14).

3.2 Drying Of The Plant Material

The cleaned and washed collected plant materials were shade dried . After drying, the material packed in polythene bags and bags were closed tightly. Whenever required, the plant materials were taken from these stocks, powdered coarsely and used for extraction.

3.3 Organoleptic Evaluation Of Powdered Crude Drugs

The crude drugs are derived from natural sources like plants, animals and minerals. It is important that they should be properly identified and characterized for their physical and chemical characteristics. So that a control on their quality could be enforced.

Organoleptic evaluation of drugs is the evaluation on the basis of morphological and sensory profile of drugs. The powdered crude drugs were evaluated for their organoleptic properties, i.e. color, taste and odor **(Table 3.1).**

PHARMACOGNOSTIC STUDY

Table 3.1: Organoleptic evaluation of selected drugs in powder form

Characteristics	*Stevia rebaudiana*	*Tinospora cordifolia*	*Triticum aestivum*
Colour	Dark green	Light green	Light green
Taste	Intensely sweet	Bitter	Characteristic
Odour	Sweetish	Characteristic	Characteristic

3.4 Physicochemical Evaluation Of Selected plant Drugs

Physicochemical evaluation of chosen drugs of *Stevia rebaudiana*, *Tinospora cordifolia* and *Triticum aesitivum* was done to establish their authenticity and purity (Table3.2).

Determination of Foreign Organic Matter

Two hundred gm of material was spread on a glass plate. The sample was observed with a magnifying glass and the foreign organic matter present in the sample was removed and after completing this exercise the drug material weighed and difference was calculated.

Moisture Content (LOD)

An far more than water in plant materials can result in microorganism growth and deterioration following reaction. Therefore, limits for the number of water ought to be set for each given stuff. This is often necessary for material, that absorbs moisture simply or deteriorates quickly within the presence of water. The wet content of a drug ought to be decreased so as to forestall decomposition of crude drug either attributable to chemical changes or microorganism contamination. LOD can be determined for material, which do not contain compounds, which are volatile at the temperature of drying.

Approximately 2 gm of sample was accurately weighed and transferred in a previously weighed weighing bottle. The bottle was stoppered loosely, placed for 30 minutes in an oven at 105°C. After drying the bottle was cooled to room temperature in a desiccator and weighed till a constant weight. With reference to air dried sample LOD was calculated. The results are given in table 3.3.

Determination of Total ash

Total ash of a vegetable drug represent its inorganic contents which represent the purity of particularly drug. Total ash was determined as per procedure of IP. Dried crude drug (2 gm) placed in antecedently weighed clean and dry oxide vessel and incline rated at a temperature not extraordinary 450°C till free from carbon that is confirmed by the white color of the ash then placed in desiccator and allowed to chill until a continuing weight obtained. the proportion of ash was calculated with relation to the air dried drug. From this total ash the acid insoluble ash and water soluble ash were determined **(I.P.1996).**

Acid Insoluble Ash

Boiled total ash with hydrochloric acid for 5 minutes then filtered, insoluble matter was collected, washed with hot water, ignited, cooled in a dessicator and weighed. The percentage of acid insoluble ash was calculated with reference to air dried drug **(I.P. 1996)**

Water-soluble ash:

Water soluble ash is that the calculated distinction in weight between the whole ash and also the residue remaining when treatment of the whole ash with water. The whole ash was stewed with twenty five millilitre of water for five minutes and filtered through ashless paper. The residue collected on the paper was washed with hot H2O. The paper was allowed to dry and lit for quarter-hour at 450°C. the load of insoluble ash was resolute and deducted from the whole ash taken to get the water soluble ash. the proportion of water soluble ash was calculated with respect to air dried sample.

Table 3.2: Physicochemical Evaluation of *Stevia rebaudiana*, *Tinospora cordifolia* and *Triticum aestivum*

Parameter	*S. rebaudiana* (Leaves) (Values: % w/w)	*T. cordifolia* (Stems and leaves) (Values: % w/w)	*T. aestivum* (Leaves) (Values: % w/w)
Foreign organic matter	0.13±0.42	0.14±0.16	0.11±0.14
Moisture Content	9.80±1.21	8.67±1.28	11.21±1.23
Total ash	9.64±1.46	11.17 ± 1.98	10.83 ± 1.68
Acid insoluble ash	2.82±0.36	2.64 ± 0.12	3.50 ± 0.42
Water soluble ash	1.84 ± 0.08	1.20 ± 0.09	2.78 ± 0.06

3.5 Extraction of Plant Materials

Dried and coarsely powdered *S. rebaudiana*, *T. cordifolia* and *T. aestivum* were subjected for successive solvent extraction using Soxhlation method. On the basis of solvent polarity index (PI), the powdered herbal drugs were encompassed from non-polar to polar order which ensure complete extraction of phytoconstituents from plants cellular matrix **(Lorenz *et al.*, 1991)**. Following successive extraction, powdered drug was packed in Soxhlet and petroleum ether 60-80°C (PI = 0.1), chloroform (PI=4.3) and methanol (PI=6.6) was used as non-polar to polar solvent respectively.

Scheme for successive solvent extraction:

In order to successive extraction, coarsely powdered plant material was extracted with 60-80°C of petroleum ether, chloroform and methanol respectively. After first solvent treatment in order (60-80°C of petroleum ether) complete defatting was ensured, and extract was filtered and solvent recovered using recovery unit and filtrate concentrated under vacuum. Marc obtained was air dried completely and subjected to next solvent extraction using chloroform. After completion of chloroform extraction, extract was filtered and filtrate concentrated under vacuum and obtained marc was dried to remove chloroform and subjected to methanol extraction. Extracts obtained with each solvent was weighted (w/w) and percentage yield was calculated.

Table 3.3: Plant extracts and their abbreviated nomenclature

Drug	Extract	Abbreviated nomenclature
Stevia rebaudiana	Petroleum ether(60-80°C) extract	PEESR
	chloroform extract	CESR
	Methanol extract	MESR
Tinospora cordifolia	Petroleum ether(60-80°C) extract	PEETC
	chloroform extract	CETC
	Methanol extract	METC
Triticum aestivum	Petroleum ether(60-80°C) extract	PEETA
	chloroform extract	CETA
	Methanol extract	META

Table 3.4 : Polarity based successive solvent extraction and yield of derived extracts

Plant material	Extract			
	Type and extract name	Texture	Color	%Yield (w/w)
Stevia rebaudiana (Leaves)	Petroleum ether (60-80°C) Extract	Semisolid sticky mass	Light green	21.65
	Chloroform extract	Solid sticky	Dark green	8.32
	Methanol Extract	Solid sticky	Light green	60.56
Tinospora cordifolia (stems and leaves)	Petroleum ether (60-80°C) Extract	Semi solid	Brownish black	15.28
	Chloroform extract	Solid	Dark brown	11.4
	Methanol Extract	Semi solid	Light Brown	57.73
Triticum aestivum (leaves)	Petroleum ether (60-80°C) Extract	Solid	Light brown	9.85
	Chloroform extract	Semi solid	Dark brown	12.74
	Methanol Extract	Semi solid	Light brown	66.58

PRELIMINARY ANTIDIABETIC SCREENING OF EXTRACTS

4.1 In vitro methods

Glucose absorption retarded by inhibition of the carbohydrate hydrolyzing enzymes α-amylase and α-glucosidase. α-amylase which is present in pancreatic juice is responsible for breaking of starch into absorbable molecules, maltose(**Gupta R et al, 2003**). α-glucosidase, present in intestine play role in carbohydrate digestion (**Anam K et al, 2009**). Both of these enzymes inhibitors retarded process of saccharide breakdownwithin the bowel and reduce the postprandial blood glucose levels. (**Bakırel T et al, 2008 and Fred-Jaiyesimi A et al, 2009**).

Chemicals

The α-amylase and α-Glucosidasewere bought from Sigma-Aldrich. Chemicals like 3, 5-Dinitro salicylic acid, sodium potassium tartarate, sodium chloride and sodium hydroxide were obtained from Himedia, Mumbai. Chemicals used in present investigation were of analytical grades.

4.1.1 *In-vitro* Alpha-Amylase inhibition assay

α-amylase repressive activity was studied by enzyme-starch system. Sample mixed with potato starch (1% and 4% respectively), incubated for one hour at 37 °C after adding α-amylase (100 mg). centrifuged for 15 min (3,000 rpm) after adding 2ml of sodium hydroxide then glucose was estimated. A control test was also done without addition of test sample (**Ou S et al 2001**).

% Inhibition = Absorbance of control – Absorbance of test/Absorbance of control X100

IC_{50} (concentration of extract required to inhibit 50% of PPA) values of Acarbose and extracts were determined from graphs of percentage inhibition versus concentration (μg/ml).

PRELIMINARY ANTIDIABETIC SCREENING OF EXTRACTS

4.1.2 In-*vitro* α-Glucosidase inhibition assay

50 μl α-glucosidase (1.0 U/ml) incubated with various extracts (100 μl) at 37°C for 10 min. 50 μl of *p*-nitrophenyl-α-D glucopyranoside (5 mM) used as reaction initiater. All solutions were prepared in 0.1 M phosphate buffer. P-nitrophenol'sdynamics were measured spectrophotometrically at 405 nm. (**Rao et al., 2009**).

.% Inhibition = Absorbance of control − Absorbance of test/Absorbance of control X100

where Ac and Ae are the absorbance of the control and extract respectively. As controlAcarbose was used.

In-vitro α-amylaseandα-glucosidasesinhibitory activity data of Acarbose are given in. Table-4.1. *In-vitro* α-amylaseinhibitory activity of different extracts of *S. rebaudiana*, *T. cordifolia*and *T. aestivum* data are given in Table-4.2, Table-4.3and Table-4.4 respectively. *In-vitro* α-glucosidasesinhibitory activity data of *S. rebaudiana, T. cordifolia*and *T. aestivum* are given in Table-4.5, Table-4.6 and Table-4.7.

Table 4.1.The percentage inhibition of α-amylase and α-glucosidase by Acarbose.

S. No	Concentration (μg/ml)	% Inhibition of α-amylase	% Inhibition of α-glucosidase
1.	20	32.15	29.12
2.	40	56.64	42.16
3.	60	71.20	61.28
4.	80	94.36	69.3
5.	100	106.40	78.54
6.	IC50	36.22	50.43

PRELIMINARY ANTIDIABETIC SCREENING OF EXTRACTS

Table 4.2. The percentage inhibition of α-amylase by SR extracts

S. No	Concentration (µg/ml)	% Inhibition of alpha amylase		
		PEESR	CESR	MESR
1.	20	11.46	00	30.36
2.	40	16.32	2.80	2.80
3.	60	21.54	5.72	37.82
4.	80	28.42	6.54	48.20
5.	100	32.78	10.24	56.16
6.	IC50	163.83	559.87	84.63

Table 4.3. The percentage inhibition of α-amylase by TC extracts

S. No	Concentration (µg/ml)	% Inhibition of alpha amylase		
		PEETC	CETC	METC
1.	20	20.10	16.85	51.24
2.	40	22.54	19.42	68.62
3.	60	26.72	22.64	80.46
4.	80	33.48	25.98	93.52
5.	100	38.50	27.56	102.38
6.	IC50	151.51	258.34	14.03

Table 4.4. The percentage inhibion of α-amylase by TA extracts

S. No	Concentration (µg/ml)	% Inhibition of alpha amylase		
		PEETA	CETA	META
1.	20	3.38	1.18	38.98
2.	40	7.26	5.12	55.25
3.	60	12.68	9.23	68.04
4.	80	18.30	15.38	79.22
5.	100	21.45	32.57	86.26
6.	IC50	219.32	162.24	33.8

PRELIMINARY ANTIDIABETIC SCREENING OF EXTRACTS

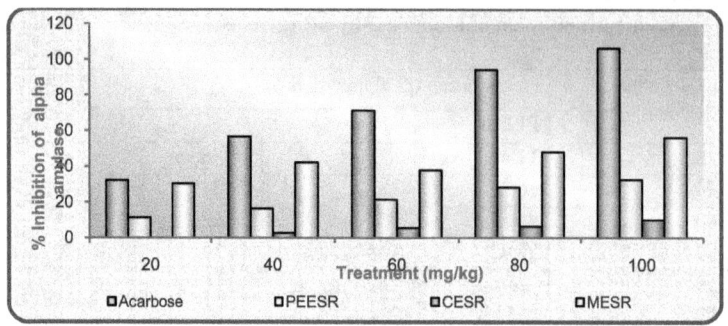

Graph: 4.1 α-amylase inhibition by extracts of *S. rebaudiana* in comparision with acarbose

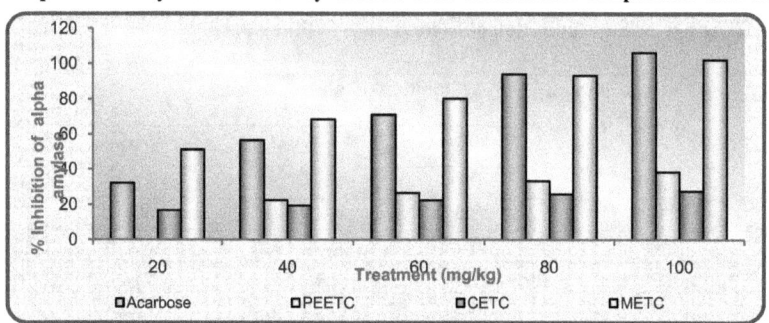

Graph: 4.2 α-amylase inhibition by extracts of *T. cordifolia* in comparision with acarbose

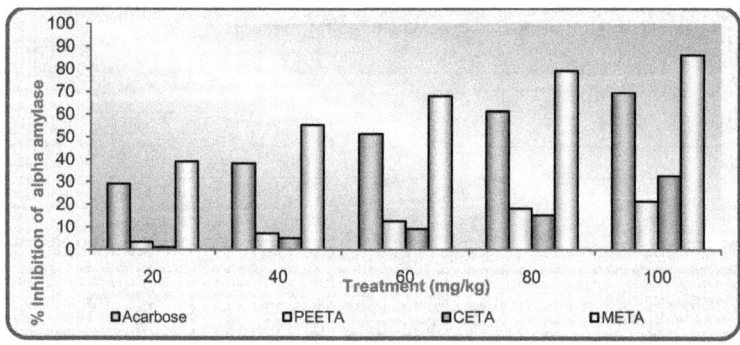

Graph: 4.3 α-amylase inhibition by extracts of *T. aestivum* in comparision with acarbose

PRELIMINARY ANTIDIABETIC SCREENING OF EXTRACTS

Table 4.5 The percentage inhibition α-glucosidase by different extracts of *S. rebaudiana*

S. No	Concentration (µg/ml)	% Inhibition of alpha glucosidases		
		PEESR	CESR	MESR
1.	20	11.94	00.00	18.46
2.	40	14.20	1.12	25.50
3.	60	18.54	6.80	37.82
4.	80	24.70	10.26	42.35
5.	100	29.65	13.73	58.80
6.	IC50	192.01	298.35	87.62

Table 4.6 The percentage inhibition of α-glucosidase by TC extracts

S. No	Concentration (µg/ml)	% Inhibition of alpha glucosidase		
		PEETC	CETC	METC
1.	20	18.92	11.52	35.34
2.	40	25.74	19.26	56.67
3.	60	31.20	23.20	68.50
4.	80	36.00	28.14	76.72
5.	100	39.64	33.56	82.45
6.	IC50	136.47	161.94	35.64

Table 4.7 The percentage inhibition of α-glucosidase by TA extracts

S. No	Concentration (µg/ml)	% Inhibition of alpha glucosidase		
		PEETA	CETA	META
1.	20	10.16	8.62	26.50
2.	40	15.08	12.54	33.91
3.	60	21.37	18.25	41.64
4.	80	28.46	23.38	52.36
5.	100	32.55	30.15	62.70
6.	IC50	158.36	176.88	74.54

PRELIMINARY ANTIDIABETIC SCREENING OF EXTRACTS

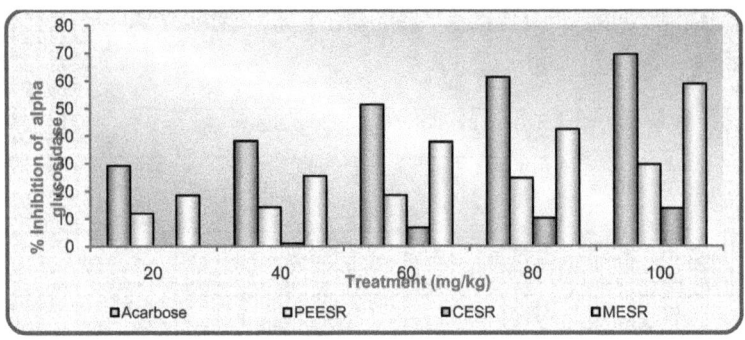

Graph: 4.4 α-glucosidase inhibition by of *S. rebaudiana* extracts in comparision with acarbose

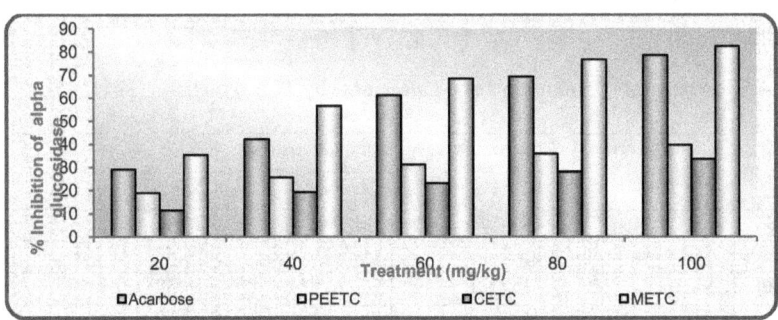

Graph: 4.5 α-glucosidase inhibition by extracts of *T. cordifolia* in comparision with acarbose

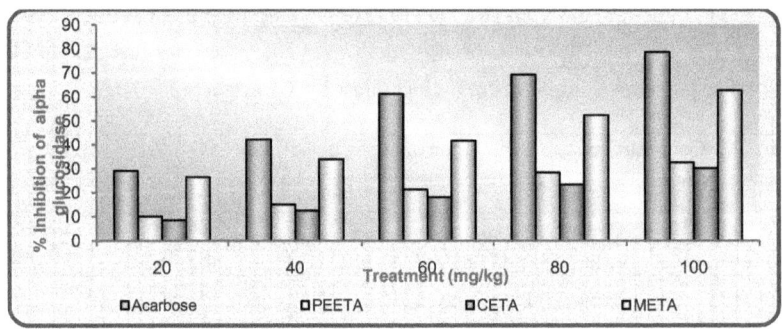

Graph: 4.6 α-glucosidase inhibition by extracts of *T. aestivum* in comparision with acarbose

PRELIMINARY ANTIDIABETIC SCREENING OF EXTRACTS

4.2. In vivo methods : Acute Toxicity Studies

For allocation of different groups of animals and prior to commencement of antidiabetic study, LD_{50} of extracts was decided.

4.2.1. Selection of animals:

Albino rats were selectedand housed in well-ventilated rooms polypropylene cageswith proper availability of water and rat pellet feed.

4.2.2 Preparation of drugs samples:

Extracts were prepared as 2%gum acacia suspensions. These were administrated through the oral route.

4.2.3 LD_{50} determination:

Acute toxic studies were conducted to determine safe dose by an up and down staircase method as described by **Ghosh (1984)**. The test substances were administered in a single-dose orally to over night fasted animals by gavage. Three animals were used in each category and starting dose lied in the range of 2000-5000 mg/kg body weight (**OECD guideline 423**). 1/10thof the lethal dose was used as effective dose for antidiabetic screening where 5, 10 and 20 times of the effective dose of extracts and fractions were optimized. After administration the animals were observed continuously for 1 hr for the next 4 hrs and then upto 24 hrs for Behavioral, Neurologica and Autonomic profile(**Turner, 1965**).After a period of 24 and 72 h mice were observed for lethality or death, if any. Animals were given water *ad libitum* and were fed with rat pellet feed (Hindustan lever Ltd Mumbai, India)and were given 5% glucose solution to drink over-night to counter hypoglycemic shock. The experimental protocol was approved by Institutional Animal Ethics Committee (Reg. No.1169/ac/08/CPCSEA) and animal care was taken as per the guidelines of Committee for the Purpose of Control and Supervision of Experiments on Animals (CPCSEA).Albino mice of either sex weighing 20-30 gm were selected. They were individually housed in polypropylene cages, in well-ventilated rooms, under hygienic condition.

PRELIMINARY ANTIDIABETIC SCREENING OF EXTRACTS

Table 4.8 : Acute toxicity study of crude extracts

S.No.	Crude Extracts	LD_{50} Cut-off (mg/kg body weight)
1.	PEESR	2000
2.	CESR	2000
3.	MESR	2000
4.	PEESR	2000
5.	CETC	2000
6.	METC	2000
7.	PEETA	2000
8.	CETA	2000
9.	META	2000

4.3 Antidiabetic Screening models

4.3.1 Albino rats were selectedand housed in well-ventilated rooms polypropylene cageswith proper availability of water and rat pellet feed.

4.3.2 Standard drug and chemicals:

All Chemical used for research work bought Streptozotocin and glybenclamide were purchased from Sigma Chemical Co. (USA). Kits for Lipid profile,Total protein, Albumin,Creatinin and Urea, and Enzyme linked immunosorbent assay were purchased from Erba Diagnostics, Mannheim.

4.3.3 Administration of dosage:

The extracts were suspended in 2% Acacia. Dose was calculated as 100,200 and 400mg/kg body weight and given orally using stainless steel canula observing that volume of drug solution administered did not exceeded 2ml.

PRELIMINARY ANTIDIABETIC SCREENING OF EXTRACTS

4.3.4 Statistical Analysis of Experimental Data

All the experimental data for statistical analysis were presented as mean± SEM. One-way analysis of variance (ANOVA) was applied by Dunnett's test and calculated the statistical significance in case of multiple comparisions with control groups only. For dependent variables (before and after the treatment) paired student's

All biochemical estimations were recorded as Mean ± S.E. Data were analyzed by one way analysis of variance (ANOVA) and Dunnett's test.

Blood sampling and glucose estimation:

For blood glucose determination, blood was withdrawn by tail snipping technique (Aydin*et al.*, 1994).

Blood glucose:

One Touch Glucometer (Accu-Check Sensor, Roche Diagnostics, Germany) used for Blood glucose was estimation. Glucose determination based on the concept that in the presence of glucose oxidase, glucose and the oxygen reactwith each other and produce gluconic acid and H_2O_2 subsequently. Produced H_2O_2 turns dye blue in a presence of peroxidase. Glucometer is suitable diagnostically in term of test accuracy, where a drop of blood is sufficient to get the results and easy to access at ambient temperature >95° F and hence used.

4.4 ACUTE STUDY : Single Dose One Day Treatment

4.4.1 Effect of extracts on blood glucose in normal fasted rats:

Different groups of rats were allocated (contain 6 rats each) to normal control (vehicle treated), standard (GLB) and plants extracts (*S.rebaudiana, T.cordifolia*and *T. aestivum*) treated groups

The rats were fasted over-night (18 h) and their fasting BG estimated. For normal control group only vehicle was given whereas for standard and treated (extract) groups were fed to GLB and extracts (100, 200, 400 mg/kg, p.o.). After treatment of all groups of

PRELIMINARY ANTIDIABETIC SCREENING OF EXTRACTS

rats, blood glucose was determined at 0, 2, 4 and 6 h interval. Estimation of BG was carried out by tail snipping method for which One Touch Glucometer was used and observations were recorded **(Table 4.9; Graph 4.7, Table 4.10; Graph 4.8 and Table 4.11, Graph 4.9).**

Table 4.9 : Effect of *S. rebaudiana* extracts on BG level in normal fasted rats

S. No.	Treatment (mg/kg)	Blood glucose (mg/dl)			
		0h (FBG)	2h	4h	6h
1.	NC	87.10±1.52	87.52±1.31	87.24±2.06	87.42±1.74
2.	PEESR100	88.54±2.02	87.90±1.84	88.14±1.84	88.10±1.60
3.	PEESR200	88.10±2.25	88.46±1.34	88.15±2.62	88.20±2.54
4.	PEESR400	88.00±2.58	87.80±1.62	87.58±1.40	87.46±1.98
5.	CESR100	87.32±1.92	86.94±1.50	86.22±1.81	86.02±2.06
6.	CESR200	89.07±1.80	89.20±2.86	89.10±2.30	89.21±1.10
7.	CESR400	88.02±1.60	88.15±1.65	87.48±2.42	87.50±2.03
8.	MESR100	87.74±2.10	87.14±1.92	86.60±2.32	77.50±1.34 [a b]
9.	MESR200	86.58±1.88	84.70±1.26	76.52 [a b] ±1.86	76.10±1.82 [a b]
10.	MESR400	88.36±2.04	85.20±1.50	79.48 [a b] ±1.84	78.14±2.08 [a b]
11.	GLB0.3	88.24±1.92	86.82±1.72	80.44 [a b] ±2.01	74.60±1.84 [a b]

PRELIMINARY ANTIDIABETIC SCREENING OF EXTRACTS

Table 4.10 : Effect of *T.cordifolia* extracts on blood glucose level in normal fasted rats

S. No.	Treatment (mg/kg)	Blood glucose (mg/dl)			
		0 h (FBG)	2h	4h	6h
1.	NC	87.10±1.52	87.52±1.31	87.24±2.06	87.42±1.74
2.	PETC100	87.34±2.34	90.1±2.03	88±2.16	87.16±2.08
3.	PETC200	88.09±2.18	88.74±2.40	90.18±2.86	89.33±3.12
4.	PETC400	86.16±2.56	85.14±1.88	82.25±2.00	84.16±1.48
5.	CETC100	82.46±3.20	82.11±2.32	81.76±3.16	82.12±2.64
6.	CETC200	83.78±2.75	84.06±2.98	83.94±2.79	83.90±3.19
7.	CETC400	88.60±3.43	88.23±3.02	87.32±3.65	87.94±2.00
8.	METC100	82.48±3.10	81.20±2.76	80.23±1.54	72.50±3.14 a b
9.	METC200	82.75±2.72	80.41±2.82	74.62±2.91 a b	67.40±1.83 a b
10	METC400	86.26±2.10	82.05±3.16	72.46±2.87a b	66.27±1.87 a b
11.	GLB0.3	88.24±1.92	86.82±1.72	79.44 a b ±2.01	71.60±1.84 a b

PRELIMINARY ANTIDIABETIC SCREENING OF EXTRACTS

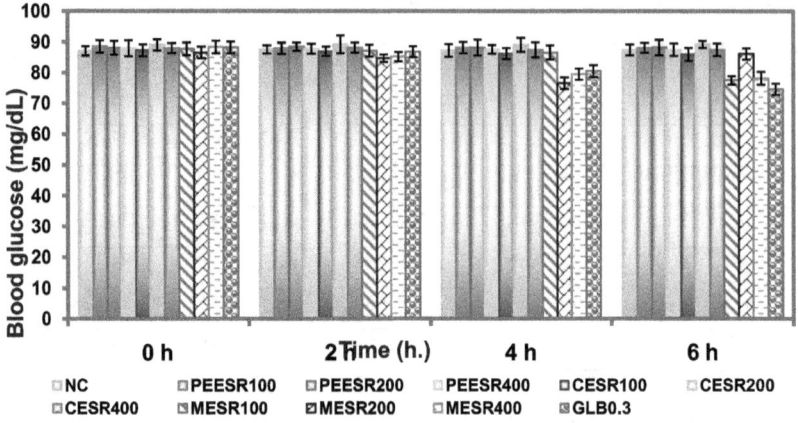

Graph 4.7 : Effect of *S. rebaudiana* extracts on blood glucose level in normal fasted rats

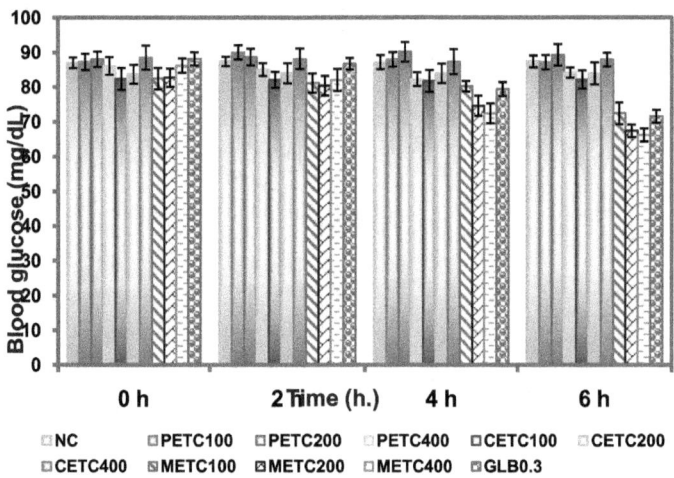

Graph 4.8 : Effect of *T.cordifolia* extracts on blood glucose level in normal fasted rats

PRELIMINARY ANTIDIABETIC SCREENING OF EXTRACTS

Table 4.11: Effect of *T. aestivum* extracts on blood glucose level in normal fasted rats

S. No.	Treatment (mg/kg)	Blood glucose (mg/dl)			
		0 h ((FBG)	2h	4h	6h
1.	NC	87.10±1.52	87.52±1.31	87.24±2.06	87.42±1.74
2.	$PETA_{100}$	92.74±1.26	95.30±2.37	93.30±2.21	92.26 ±1.26
3.	$PETA_{200}$	94.10±2.58	93.32±1.98	95.28 ±2.74	94.43±2.92
4.	$PETA_{400}$	91.20±2.05	90.24±1.62	89.90±1.52	89.26±1.54
5.	$CETA_{100}$	93.26±2.14	92.48±1.64	92.00±1.55	92.60±1.55
6.	$CETA_{200}$	94.20±2.44	93.36±1.36	93.50±1.72	92.39±1.17
7.	$CETA_{400}$	91.70±2.50	89.20±1.33	91.30±2.52	90.44±1.93
8.	$META_{100}$	90.40±2.34	93.40±1.35	94.03±2.19	94.25±2.17
9.	$META_{200}$	93.07±1.26	92.20±2.26	93.50±2.42	91.30±1.22
10	$META_{400}$	90.37±1.19	94.19±1.88	92.30±2.51	91.40±2.32
11.	GLB	88.24±1.92	86.82±1.72	79.44 ±2.01 [a b]	71.60±1.84 [a b]

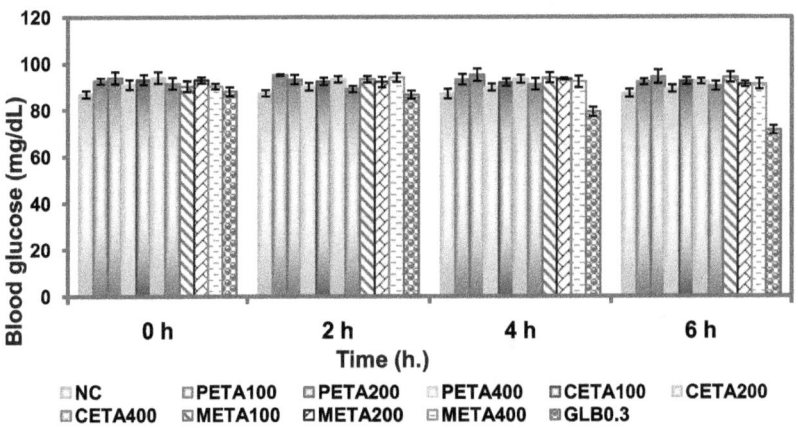

Graph 4.9 : Effect of *T. Aestivum* extracts on blood glucose level in normal fasted rats

4.3.2 Effect of extracts on OGTT in normal fasted rats

PRELIMINARY ANTIDIABETIC SCREENING OF EXTRACTS

OGTT provides the information regarding severity of diabetes mellitus and known as 'gold standard' for its diagnosis. It is a useful epidemiological tool and has been used to determine the prevalence of diabetes. For OGTT assessment, overnight **(Kumar et al., 2006)**. 50% Glucose solution (2 ml) was administered to test the Glucose tolerance. The animals were pretreated ½ hour before with the extracts to be tested. All the extracts were prepared as a suspension by triturating with 2% Gum acacia 16hr. fasted animals in control group received glucose (1g/kg, p.o.) and blood glucose was determined at 0, 1/2, 1 and 2 h after, using glucometer. The standard treated, extracts treated and fractions treated groups first received GLB as a standard drug, crude extracts and their fractions (400, 200, 100 mg/kg, p.o.) and two hour later glucose (1g/kg, p.o.) was fed. The blood glucose determined likewise to previous manner.

The dose was given using a syringe needle, which was grated and softened at the tip (to avoid any injury to the animals). . Animals were observed for 3 hours at regular intervals after the administration of test extracts. In all cases, no death was observed within 24 hours. **(Table 4.12, Graph 4.10, Table 4.13, Graph 4.11 and Table 4.14, Graph 4.12).**

Table 4.12 : Effect of SR extracts on OGTT in normal fasted Rats

PRELIMINARY ANTIDIABETIC SCREENING OF EXTRACTS

S. No.	Treatment (mg/kg)	Blood glucose (mg/dl)			
		0 h (FBG)	1/2 h	1 h	2 h
1.	NC + Glucose	87.28±1.22	162.56±5.26	94.16±2.50	89.16±2.97
2.	$PEESR_{100}$ + Glucose	82.40±2.45	164.10±4.40	137.18±3.03	90.45±3.01
3.	$PEESR_{200}$ + Glucose	83.34±3.04	160.20±7.12	138.48±2.50	89.74±3.52
4.	$PEESR_{400}$ + Glucose	86.50±2.84	168.8±5.56	150.28±5.01	90.25±2.82
5.	$CESR_{100}$ + Glucose	88.32±2.04	168.78±4.62	139.30±3.82	91.10±3.03
6.	$CESR_{200}$ + Glucose	85.10±3.02	165.10±5.04	130.05±3.96	90.77±2.04
7.	$CESR_{400}$ + Glucose	82.63±1.72	175.64±5.05	132.22±4.10	88.84±3.04
8.	$MESR_{100}$ + Glucose	84.25±3.43	134.20±4.46[a]	124.80±6.10	95.14±7.04
9.	$MESR_{200}$ + Glucose	89.62±2.98	132.80±6.10[a]	122.60±6.34	91.20±4.24
10.	$MESR_{400}$ + Glucose	86.14±1.94	120.20±4.82[a]	116.80±4.20	90.60±6.10
11.	GLB + Glucose	89.36±2.20	103.20±3.18[a]	94.82±2.50	90.76±3.26

Table 4.13 : Effect of TC extracts on OGTT in normal fasted rats

S. No.	Treatment	Blood glucose (mg/dl)

PRELIMINARY ANTIDIABETIC SCREENING OF EXTRACTS

	(mg/kg)	0 h (FBG)	1/2 h	1 h	2 h
1.	NC + Glucose	87.28±1.34	162.56±5.26	94.16±2.50	89.16±2.97
2.	PEETC100 + Glucose	86.08±2.96	168.14±4.64	136.87±3.82	97.48±3.01
3.	PEETC200 + Glucose	88.44±2.50	170.70±4.64	135.00±3.90	95.42±2.06
4.	PEETC400 + Glucose	81.24±2.67	163.25±4.08	134.25±4.02	98.00±3.46
5.	CETC100 + Glucose	82.28±3.12	158.88±3.86	127.43±2.60	96.47±3.00
6.	CETC200 + Glucose	80.30±2.38	164.25±2.68	136.35±5.00	96.56±2.80
7.	CETC400+ Glucose	81.21±1.28	150.22±2.35	132.20±4.80	92.20±3.20
.8.	MEC100+ Glucose	82.28±3.12	126.38±4.86 a	117.43±2.68	90.47±3.30
9.	METC200 + Glucose	82.34±2.05	110.78±3.30a	105.12±2.06	85.78±3.02
10	METC400 + Glucose	80.50±1.35	98.34±5.78a	86.17±1.20	84.35±2.37
11.	GLB + Glucose	89.36±2.20	103.20±3.18a	94.82±2.50	90.76±3.26

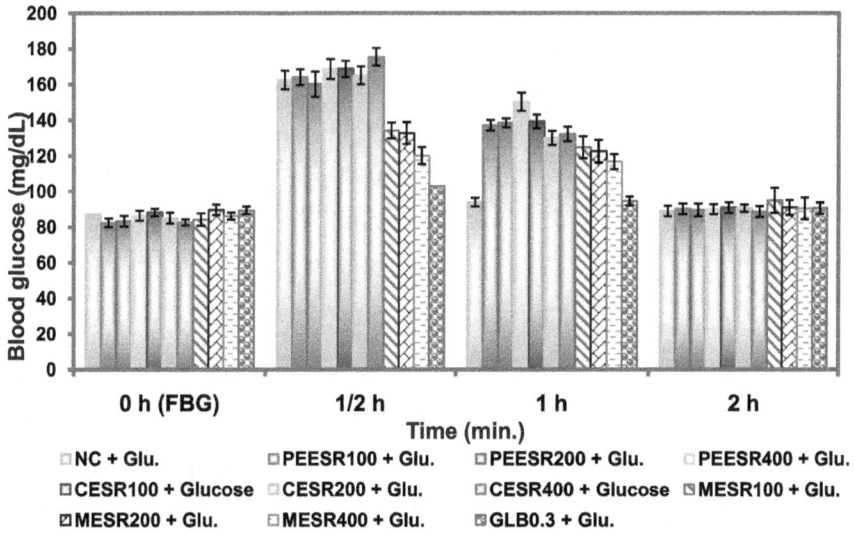

Graph 4.10: Effect of SR extracts on OGTT in normal fasted Rat

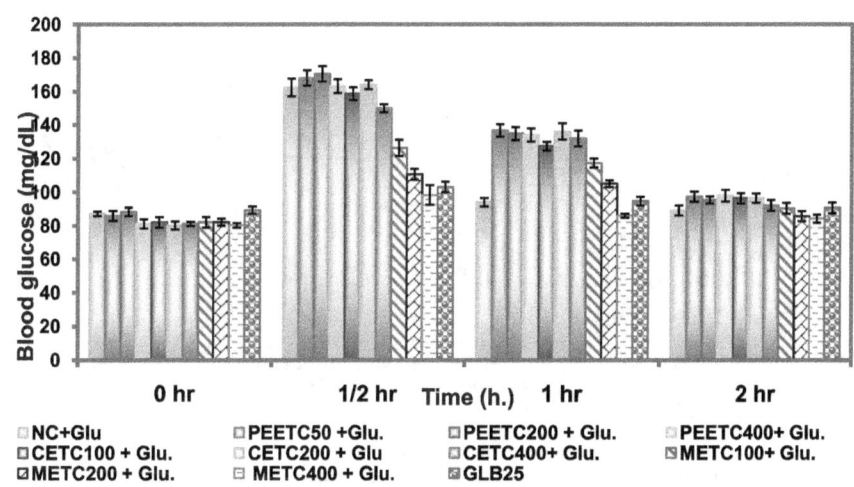

Graph 4.11: Effect of TC extracts on OGTT in normal fasted Rats

PRELIMINARY ANTIDIABETIC SCREENING OF EXTRACTS

Table 4.14 : Effect of TA extracts on OGTT in normal fasted rats

S. No.	Treatment (mg/kg)	Blood glucose (mg/dl)			
		0 h (FBG)	1/2 h	1 h	2 h
1.	NC + Glucose	87.28±1.34	162.56±5.26	94.16±2.50	89.16±2.97
2.	PEETA$_{100}$ + Glucose	89.36±2.68	166.10±5.24	149.24±4.98	98.62±2.40
3.	PEETA$_{200}$ + Glucose	88.41±2.94	173.16±5.80	140.28±3.52	96.28±3.38
4.	PEETA$_{400}$ + Glucose	90.18±3.24	169.18±4.35	131.06±2.54	93.05±2.32
5.	CETA$_{100}$ + Glucose	89.12±3.67	170.14±3.21	158.28±4.14	100.18±1.20
6.	CETA$_{200}$ + Glucose	91.54±1.63	172.86±4.30	144.28±3.86	105.28±3.80
7.	CETA$_{400}$ + Glucose	90.34±2.44	169.15±4.89	140.40±5.04	102.07±4.80
8.	META$_{100}$ + Glucose	88.12±2.26	125.24±4.03 a	104.16±3.28	97.10±3.52
9.	META$_{200}$ + Glucose	90.76±3.98	104.33±4.87 a	96.6±2.50	90.77±2.68
10	META$_{400}$ + Glucose	92.57±2.30	107.09±4.36 a	91.02±3.52	88. ±2.544
11.	GLB + Glucose	89.36±2.20	103.20±3.18a	94.82±2.50	90.76±3.26

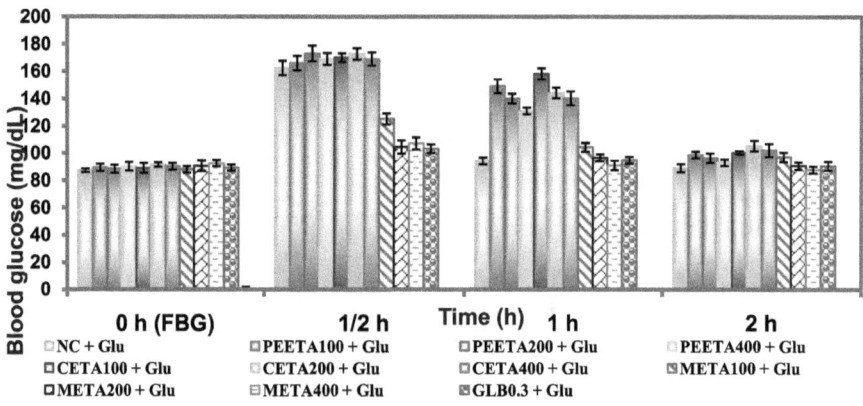

Graph 4.12: Effect of TA extracts on OGTT in normal fasted Rats

4.3.3 Effect of extracts on BG level in streptozotocin-induced diabetic rats

PRELIMINARY ANTIDIABETIC SCREENING OF EXTRACTS

For preliminary antidiabetic study of the crude extracts, streptozotocin was used as a diabetogenic agent. The rats were made diabetic by intraperitoneal injection of fresh solution of streptozotocin (45mg/kg, b.w.) in 0.1 M citrate buffer, in overnight fasted condition.Due to instability of STZ in aqueousmedia, before use it's solution is prepared in citrate buffer (pH 4.5). then allowed a rest period of 2 days with free access of food and water **(Brosky and Logothelopoulos, 1969)**. BG level, determined at 72 h and then on day 7 after streptozotocini.p. injection. During the animal allocation for antidiabetic screening, animal those having blood glucose level above 250 mg/kg, were allocated for antidiabetic screening, containing six animals in eavery group. During study BG of treated groupsi.e.control and crude extracts (100, 200, 400 mg/kg) were taken at 0, 2, 4, 6 h and estimated using glucometer.**(Table 4.15; Graph 4.13 and Table 4.16; Graph 4.14 and Table 4.15; Graph 4.15).**

Table 4.15 : Effect of *S.rebaudiana* extracts on BG level in STZ-induced diabetic rats

S. No.	Treatment (mg/kg)	Blood glucose (mg/dl)			
		0 h (FBG)	2 h	4 h	6 h
1.	DC	291±11.62	294.16±8.56	290.08±11.62	292.24±10.58
2.	PEESR$_{100}$	277.87±9.66	281.44±11.62	278.62±10.58	279.34±9.14
3.	PEESR$_{200}$	280±11.02	279.12±10.8	277.18±9.66	277.33±12.26
4.	PEESR$_{400}$	274.7±9.38	274.16±12.53	272.03±10.45	270.07±11.90
5.	CESR$_{100}$	267.4±11.62	266.09±10.58	265.55±8.56	262.12±8.56
6.	CESR$_{200}$	271.06±11.56	272.20±9.03	271.33±10.62	270.48±10.50
7.	CESR$_{400}$	270.15±8.25	271.32±10.72	270.74±8.44	268.10±11.22
8.	MESR$_{100}$	269.10±9.62	263.77±10.24	254.10±9.25^{ab}	244.00±12.17^{ab}
9.	MESR$_{200}$	286.10±7.64	279.03±8.52	243.18±6.62^{ab}	227.20±6.27^{ab}
10.	MESR$_{400}$	275.22±8.86	266.18±10.90^{ab}	238.15±5.58^{ab}	203.70±4.86^{ab}
11.	GLB	280.40±9.88	273.09±8.56	223.55±9.72^{ab}	195.12±7.44^{ab}

Table 4.16 : Effect of TCextracts on BG level in streptozotocin-induced diabetic rats

PRELIMINARY ANTIDIABETIC SCREENING OF EXTRACTS

S. No.	Treatment (mg/kg)	Blood glucose (mg/dl)			
		0 h(FBG)	2 h	4 h	6 h
1.	DC	284.42±10.18	284.12±9.52	283.74±12.20	284.18±11.15
2.	$PEETC_{100}$	288.12±11.54	289.09±12.48	287.7±9.42	286.2± 8.84
3.	$PEETC_{200}$	286.15±9.56	284.58± 8.02	285.3±12.74	284.71±11.66
4.	$PEETC_{400}$	291.16± 8.42	290.35±11.71	289.5 ±9.04	288.20±12.63
5.	$CETC_{100}$	285.98±9.94	283.4±10.72	283.66±10.25	284.02±10.25
6.	$CETC_{200}$	287.1±12.33	285.1±10.20	284.19±9.88	283.71±11.00
7.	$CETC_{400}$	290.13±9.25	288.2±9.88	285.8±11.66	286.1±10.25
8.	$METC_{100}$	284.12±9.92	283.09±11.34	267.7±8.56^{ab}	245.2±9.72^{ab}
9.	$METC_{200}$	287.50±10.66	280.58±8.70	260.3±9.72^{ab}	201.71±8.56^{ab}
10	$METC_{400}$	288.18±9.56	279.35±10.47	230.42±11.66^{ab}	189.22±9.72^{ab}
11.	$GLB_{0.3}$	270.25±8.80	261.42 ±9.15	210.28±10.04^{ab}	182.10±9.15^{ab}

PRELIMINARY ANTIDIABETIC SCREENING OF EXTRACTS

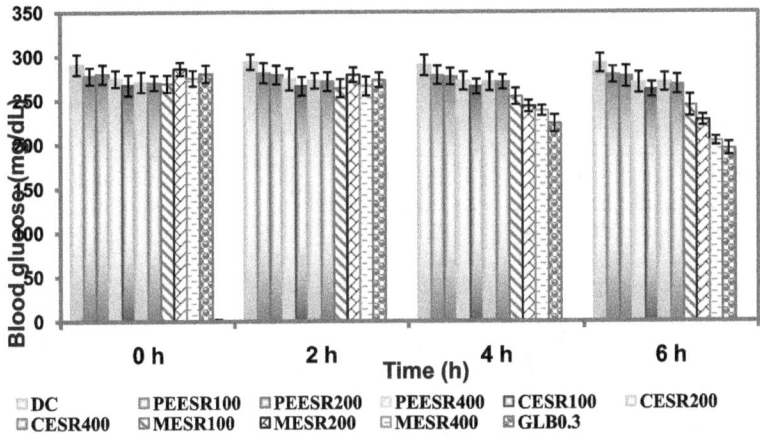

Graph 4.13 : Effect of SR extracts on BG level in streptozotocin-induced diabetic rats

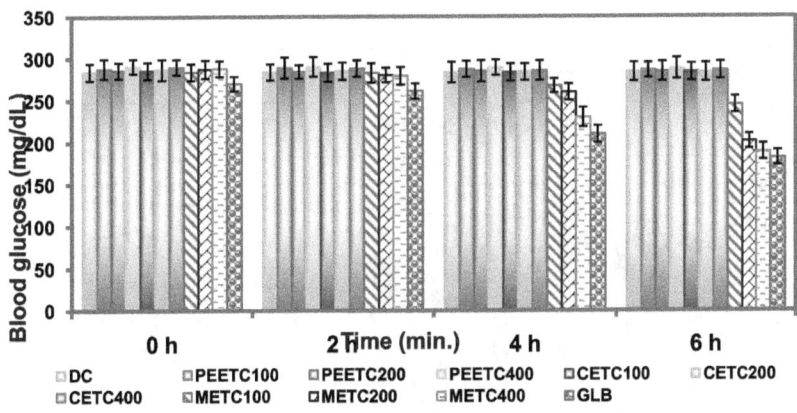

Graph 4.14: Effect of extracts of TC on BG level in streptozotocin-induced diabetic rats

Table 4.17 : Effect of TA extracts on BG level in streptozotocin-induced diabetic rats

S. No.	Treatment (mg/kg)	Blood glucose (mg/dl)			
		0 h(FBG)	2 h	4 h	6 h
1.	DC	284.02±11.98	283.78±9.45	284.03±12.75	284.21±10.40
2.	PEETA$_{100}$	280.87±9.46	279.94±11.82	280.60.±10.41	281.34±9.82
3.	PEETA$_{200}$	288.00±9.78	287.12±13.04	286.5±9.35	285.30±10.84
4.	PEETA$_{400}$	284.70±12.08	283.10±8.02	284.50±9.15	282.07±8.93
5.	CETA$_{100}$	279.92±11.22	276.26±10.09	272.65±9.08	278.00±10.45
6.	CETA$_{200}$	292.50±9.70	290.10±11.10	291.10±11.40	290.11±12.00
7.	CETA$_{400}$	283.18±8.86	281.20±13.46	282.62±10.42	280.56±11.62
8.	META$_{100}$	281.24±11.57	277.14±9.54	250.52±9.20	236.26±11.20[a b]
9.	META$_{200}$	278.85±10.42	263.58±10.56	241.30±8.68[a b]	220.54±8.26[a b]
10	META$_{400}$	275.64±9.82	252.30±8.62	230.06±8.12[a b]	218.22±6.08[a b]
11.	GLB	290.50±9.34	264.00 ±7.92	243.55±10.48[a b]	204.43±8.36[a b]

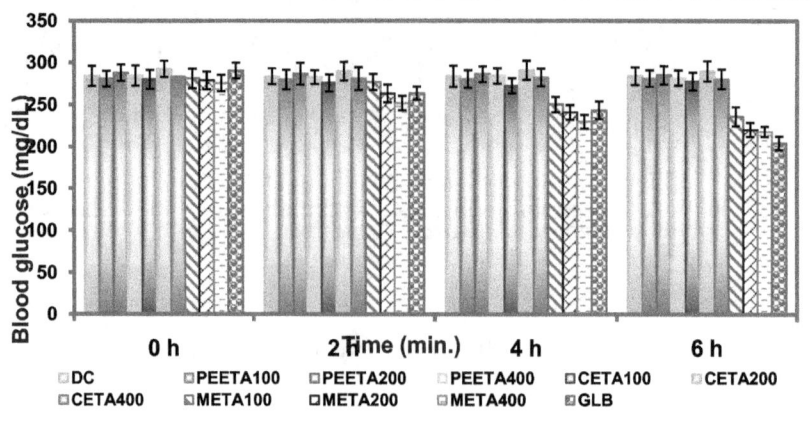

PRELIMINARY ANTIDIABETIC SCREENING OF EXTRACTS

Graph 4.15 : Effect of TA extracts on BG in streptozotocin-induced diabetic rats

4.4 Four Weeks Treatment of Extracts

On the basis of one-day single dose treatment of extracts of *S.rebaudiana, T.cordifolia* and *T. aestivum,* as their methanol extracts showed significant antidiabetic activity and hence they were selected for further study.

4.4.1 Blood glucose determination in streptozotocin-induced diabetic rats

Repeated treatment of bioactive extract of *S.rebaudiana, T.cordifolia* and *T. aestivum* using glibenclamide as a standard drug were investigated for STZ -induced diabetic rats and after two hours of last treatment, BG was estimated **(Table 4.11, Graph 4.10)**.

Table 4.18 : Effect of four weeks repeated treatment of extracts of *S.rebaudiana, T.cordifolia* and *T. aestivum* on blood glucose level in streptozotocin-induced diabetic rats

S.No.	Treatment (mg/kg)	Blood glucose level(mg/dl)	
		Before Treatment	After Treatment
1.	NC	88.46±2.31	79.10± 2.94
2.	DC	270.04±7.65	302.30± 9.25**
3.	MESR$_{200}$	261.30 ±8.22	182.52 ±7.82*
4.	METC$_{200}$	268.75 ±10.19	174.63 ± 9.26*
5.	META$_{200}$	272.24 ±8.92	180.30± 8.60*
6.	GLB	265.18±7.94	154.54± 4.01*

PRELIMINARY ANTIDIABETIC SCREENING OF EXTRACTS

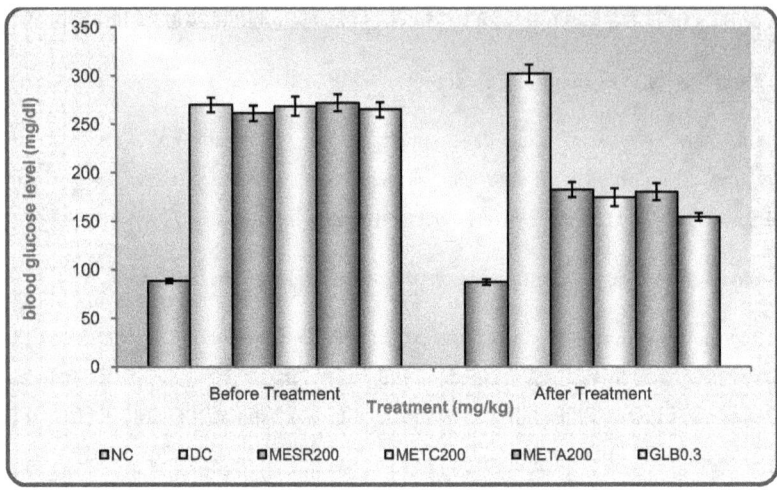

Graph 4.16: Effect of four weeks treatment of extracts of *S.rebaudiana*, *T.cordifolia* and *T. aestivum* on blood glucose level in streptozotocin-induced diabetic rats

FRACTIONATION OF EXTRACTS AND THEIR CHROMATOGRAPHIC STUDIES

5.1 FRACTIONATION OF EXTRACTS

Preliminary antidiabetic screening of different crude extract exhibited that, *S.rebaudiana, T.cordifolia* and *T. aestivum* methanol extract have potent antidiabetic activity and hence they were selected for further fractionation to pin-point the activity. On the basis of polarity index (PI), fractionation of methanol extract was done using benzene, ethyl acetate and ethanol by silica gel 60-80 mesh packed chromatographic column. Different fractions were collected. By using vacuum solvents were removed and fractions were dried with anhydrous Na_2SO_4, percentage yields (w/w) were calculated **(Table 5.1 and 5.2)**.

Table 5.1 : Extract fractions and their abbreviated nomenclature

Drug	Fraction	Abbreviated nomenclature
S. rebaudiana (SR)	Benzene fraction of MESR	BFSR
	Ethyl acetate fraction of MESR	EAFSR
	Ethanol fraction of MESR	EFSR
T. cordifolia (TC)	Benzene fraction of METC	BFTC
	Ethyl acetate fraction of METC	EAFTC
	Ethanol fraction of METC	EFTC
T. aestivum (TA)	Benzene fraction of META	BFTA
	Ethyl acetate fraction of META	EAFTA
	Ethanol fraction of META	EFTA

FRACTIONATION OF EXTRACTS AND THEIR CHROMATOGRAPHIC STUDIES

Table 5.2 : Yield of fractions of *S.rebaudiana*, *T.cordifolia* and *T. aestivum* obtained by column chromatography

Plant material	Fraction			
	Fraction Type	Texture	Color	%Yield (w/w)
Methanol extract of *S. rebaudiana* leaves(MESR)	Benzene fraction	Semisolid sticky mass	Black-brown	6.25
	Ethyl acetate fraction	Solid sticky	Dark-tan	22.48
	Ethanol fraction	Solid sticky	Light-tan	12.20
Methanol extract of *T. cordifolia*(METC)	Benzene fraction	Solid	brown	7.40
	Ethyl acetate fraction	Solid sticky	Dark brown	15.74
	Ethanol fraction	Solid	Light-Brown	45.27
Methanol extract of *T. aestivum*(META)	Benzene fraction	Solid	brown	8.60
	Ethyl acetate fraction	Solid sticky	Dark brown	12.52
	Ethanol fraction	Solid	Light-Brown	30.56

5.2 QUALITATIVE PHYTOCHEMICAL EVALUATION OF FRACTIONS

preliminary phytochemical screening of fractions were done as per **Kokate, 2002**. Small quantities of investigating fractions were dissolved in their parent solvent and were subjected for analysis using specific reagents and the observations were tabulated (**Table 5.3**).

(A) Tests for carbohydrates:

Molisch's test (For reducing sugars):

In the solution of fraction Molisch's reagent was added Purple ring at the junction confirm the presence carbohydrates.

FRACTIONATION OF EXTRACTS AND THEIR CHROMATOGRAPHIC STUDIES

Fehling test:

In the solution of fraction Fehling's A and Fehling's B solution was mixed on heating brick red precipitate, confirm the presence carbohydrates.

Benedict's test:

Solution to be tested heated with Benedict's reagent in same volume. Yellow or red appearance confirm the presence carbohydrates.

(B) Tests for glycosides:

Baljet test (For cardiac glycoside):

With sodium picrate glycoside gives yellow to orange color.

Keller-Kiliani test (For de-oxy-sugars):

with ferric chloride and sulphuric acid two layers were formed lower as reddish brown and upper as bluish green.

Borntrager's test (For anthraquinone glycoside):

Small quantity of alcoholic potassium hydroxide added in test solution, dilute with 4ml of water and filter, acidify with HCl, cool and shake well with 5ml of ether. Ether is separated and shakes with 2ml of dilute solution of ammonium hydroxide. Rose red to intense red color is produced in the aqueous layer is indicative of presence of anthraquinone glycosides.

Liebermann - Burchard test:

In test solution acetic anhydride and conc. H_2SO_4 were added, shaked and allowed to stand, bluish green lower layer confirm the presence of sterols.

(C) Tests for alkaloids:

A small portion of fractions are shaken in 5 ml of hydrochloric acid and filtered. The filtrates were separately tested with following reagents.

Dragendorff's test:

with potassium bismuth iodide orange brown precipitate indicate the presence of alkaloid.

Mayer's test:

Cream precipitate with potassium mercuric iodide confirm the presence of alkaloid.

Hager's reagent:

Alkaloid gives yellow precipitate with saturated picric acid solution

(D)   Test for terpenes / sterols:

Salkowaski test:

On shaking with Conc. H_2SO_4 gives golden yellow lower layer.

Liebermann-Burchard test:

With acetic anhydride and 1 ml of Conc. H_2SO_4 production of red color was confirm the presence of terpenes.

(E)   Tests for saponins:

Foam test:

Stable Foam produce on shaking the solution show the presence of saponins.

(F)   Test for flavonoids:

Sinoda test:

Pink color is obtained on adding 5 ml of 95% ethanol, to dry powdered fractions along with few drops Conc. HCl and 0.5 g of magnesium, in presence of flavonoids.

Zn/HCl reducing test:

magenta red color obtained with, zinc dust and few drops of HCl in presence of flavonoid.

(G) Tests for tannins:

With 2-3 ml of test solution, following color reaction is observable

Ferric chloride test:

gives dark color with ferric chloride solution show the presence of tannins.

Gelatin test:

white precipitate obtained on treating the solution with gelatin if tannins are present.

(H) Tests for Proteins

Biuret test:

blue color produce when treated with NaOH and dilute $CuSO_4$ indicate presence of protein

Table 5.3   Qualitative chemical Tests for bioactive fractions of *S.rebaudiana*, *T.cordifolia* and *T. aestivum*

[+] = Presence of chemical group, [-] = Absence of chemical group

S.No.	Tests	EAFSR	EFTC	EFTA
1.	Glycosides			
	Baljet test	−	+	−
	Keller-Kiliani test	−	+	−
	Raymond's test	−	+	+
	Borntrager's test	−	+	−
	Libermann-Burchard test	+	+	+
2.	Carbohydrates			
	Molisch's test	−	+	+
	Fehling's test	−	+	+
	Benedict's test	−	+	−
	Barfoed's test	+	+	+
3.	Alkaloids			
	Dragendorff's test	−	+	+
	Mayer's test	−	+	+
	Hager's test	−	+	+
4.	Terpenes/Sterols			
	Salkowaski test	+	+	−
	Liebermann-Burchard test	+	+	+
5.	Saponins			
	Foam test	−	−	−
6.	Flavonoids			
	Shinoda test	−	−	−
	Zn/HCl reducing test	−	−	+
7.	Tannins			
	Ferric chloride test	+		−
	Gelatin test	+		−
8.	Proteins			
	Biuret test	−	−	+

FRACTIONATION OF EXTRACTS AND THEIR CHROMATOGRAPHIC STUDIES

5.3 CHROMATOGRAPHIC STUDY OF EXTRACTS/FRACTIONS OF SELECTED PLANTS

For chromatographic fingerprinting of extracts/fractions of *S. rebaudiana, T. cordifolia* and *T. aestivum,* TLC and HPLC were performed.

TLC:

Chromatography is method used for the purification and separation of organic and inorganic substances. It is also found useful for the fractionation of complex mixture, separation of closely related compounds, such as isomers and in the isolation of unstable substances **(Sharma, 2001).**

5.3.1 Thin Layer Chromatographic Study of Extracts and Fractions (Stahl, 1969; Mukherjee.2010)

(i) Preparation and activation of TLC plates:

Silica gel G with distilled water (1:3) was triturated.spread on glass plates (10 cm x 20 cm.) allowed to air-dry, then heated at $110\text{-}120^0 C$ for one hour.

(ii) Preparation of sample solution:

Samples were dissolved in respective solvent and filtered.

(iii) Saturation of chamber:

Prepared mobile phase placed in the TLC chamber. A paper sheet was placed on the inner wall of the chamber to supply fast saturation and to stop border result. Chamber sealed by putting a glass plate at the mouth of chamber with paraffin.

(iv) Application of sample spots:

The spots of sample answer were applied with the assistance of skinny capillaries on the activated plates, at a distance of concerning one.5 cm. from rock bottom and were allowed to dry in air. the space between 2 spots was unbroken a minimum of ten millimete

5.3.2. Optimization and selection of mobile phase for TLC study

On the bases of better resolution and separation of the phytoconstituents of *T. cordifolia* and *T. aestivum*, its methanol extracts and derived ethanol fractions were optimized with various mobile phases **(Table 5.4 and 5.5)**. Similarly, for separation of the phytoconstituents of *S. rebaudiana*, its methanol extract and derived ethyl acetate fraction was optimized with various mobile phases **(Table 5.6)**. However for Co-optimization of extracts and their fractions, Chloroform: Glacialacetic acid:Cyclohexane(40:10:40) and Chloroform:Acetone: : Formic acid (50:25:10)for TC, TA and Chloroforme: Formic acid: Glacialacetic acid: Water (4:4:4:1) for SR were sorted out for better separation of phytoconstituents.

Table 5.4 : Co-optimization of mobile phase for TLC profile of *S. rebaudiana*

Mobile phase	Separation status	
	methanol extract	Ethylacetate fraction
Chloroforme:Acetone:Water (4:4:2)	No separation	No separation
Chloroforme:Acetone:Water (5:4:1)	No separation	No separation
Chloroforme: Formic acid:Water (4:4:2)	Tailing	Tailing
Chloroforme: Formic acid:Water (4:4:4)	Poor separation	Poor separation
Chloroforme: Formic acid:Glacialacetic acid: Water (4:4:1:1)	Good separation	Good separation
Chloroforme: Formic acid: Glacialacetic acid: Water (4:4:4:1)	Better separation	Better separation

Table 5.5 : Optimization of mobile phase for TLC profile of *T. cordifolia*

Mobile phase	Separation status	
	Methanol extract	Ethyl acetate fraction
Toluene: Ethylacetate: diethylamine (70:20:14)	No separation	No separation
Toluene: Ethylacetate: diethylamine (60:30:2o)	No separation	No separation
Chloroform: Ethylacetate: diethylamine (50:25:25)	No separation	No separation
Chloroform: Glacialacetic acid:Ethylacetate (50:30:20)	Tailing	Tailing
Chloroform:Glacialacetic acid:Cyclohexane(50:10:50)	Good separation	Good separation
Chloroform:Glacialacetic acid:Cyclohexane(40:10:40)	Better separation	Better separation

Table 5.6 : Optimization of mobile phase for TLC profile of *T. aestivum*

Mobile phase	Separation status	
	Methanol extract	Ethanol fraction
Chloroform: Ethylacetate (50:50)	No separation	No separation
Chloroform: Ethylacetate (80:20)	No separation	No separation
Chloroform: Ethylacetate: Water (80:20)	No separation	No separation
Chloroform:Acetone (50:50)	Tailing	Tailing
Chloroform:Acetone (75:25)	Tailing	Tailing
Chloroform:Acetone: : Formic acid (50:25:25)	Poor separation	Poor separation
Chloroform:Acetone: : Formic acid (50:25:10)	Better separation	Better separation

5.3.3 Co- TLC of *Stevia rebaudiana* MESR and its EAFSR

The MESR and EAFSR along with standard were run for Co-TLC investigations whereas prepared silica gel TLC plates were used. 100 mg of the **MESR and its EAFSR** and standards (stevioside) dissolved in ethanol to prepare samples and standards were applied on TLC plate.

Procedure:

The solvent system, Chloroforme: Formic acid: Glacialacetic acid: Water (4:4:4:1) was poured to a rectangular chromatographic glass chamber of 25 x 25 x 6 cm. The chamber was lined with a bit of paper to confirm adequate equilibrium. The spots of MESR and its EAFSR in conjunction with reference standards stevioside were applied on a TLC plate, dried placed vertical within the glass chamber. The chromatogram was developed until the solvent front migrated to concerning 10 cm. The plate was taken after marking the solvent front dried at room temperature and sprayed with Anisaldehyde-Sulphuric acid chemical agent. Rf values were calculated. The results are shown in Photograph (3.1) and Table (5.7).

Table 5.7 : TLC profile of S. rebaudiana methanol extracts and its ethyl acetate fraction

S.No.	Extract/ Fraction	Spot	R_f value
1.	Methanol extract	7	0.9, 0.8, 0.7, 0.5*, 0.4, 0.31, 0.1
2.	Ethyl acetate fraction	2	0.68, 0.5*

$^*R_f$ value matched with reference standard ; Stevioside

5.3.5 Co-TLC of *T. cordifolia* methanol extract and its ethanol fraction

The methanol extract and its ethanol fraction along with standard were run for Co-TLC investigation whereas prepared silica gel TLC plates were used. 100 mg of the methanol extract, its ethanol fraction and standard (berberine) was dissolved in ethanol. Prepared samples and standard was applied on TLC plate.

Procedure:

The solvent system, Chloroform: Glacialacetic acid:Cyclohexane(40:10:40) was poured in a chromatographic glass chamber of 25 x 25 x 6 cm. The chamber was lined with a bit of paper to confirm adequate equilibrium. The spots of METC and its EFTC in conjunction with reference standards berberin were applied on a TLC plate, dried placed vertical within the glass chamber. The chromatogram was developed until the solvent front migrated to concerning 10 cm. The plate was taken after marking the solvent front dried at room temperature and sprayed with Dragendorff's chemical agent. Rf values were calculated. The results are shown in. The results are given in Table (5.8) and Photograph (5.2).

Table 5.8 : TLC profile of T. cordifolia methanol extract and its ethanol fraction

S.No.	Extract/ Fraction	Spot	R_f value
1.	Methanol extract	4	0.8, 0.75, 0.65, 0.55*
2.	Ethanol fraction	2	0.8, 0.75*

* R_f Value matched with reference standard; berberine

5.3.4 Co-TLC of *T. aestivum* methanol extract and its Ethanol fraction

The methanol extract and its ethanol fraction along with standard were run for Co-TLC investigation whereas prepared silica gel TLC plates were used.100 mg of the methanol extract, its ethyl acetate fraction and standard (quercetin) were dissolved in ethanol. Samples were prepared and standard was applied on TLC plate.

Procedure:

The solvent system, Chloroform:Acetone: : Formic acid (50:25:10) was poured in a chromatographic glass chamber of 25 x 25 x 6 cm. The chamber was lined with a piece of filter paper to ensure adequate equilibrium and spots of methanolic extract, its ethyl acetate fraction and standard compound were applied on a silica gel 60 F_{254} plate. The applied spots were dried at room temperature and the plate was gently placed inside the glass chamber. The chromatogram was developed till the solvent front migrated to about 12.0 cm. The plate was taken out and solvent front was marked. The plate was dried at room temperature and sprayed anisaldehide-H_2SO_4 acid reagent. The spots (purple) developed on the plate were marked, observed under UV matched with external standard and their R_f values were calculated. The results are given in **Table (5.9)** and **Photograph (5.3)**.

Table 5.9 : TLC profile of *T. aestivum* methanol extract and its Ethanol fraction

S.No.	Extract/ fraction	Spot	R_f value
1.	Methanol extract	9	0.92, 0.78, 0.7, 0.63, 0.54*, 0.44, 0.35, 0.23, 0.05*
2.	Ethanol fraction	6	0.92, 0.78, 0.54*, 0.35, 0.23, 0.05*

*R_f Value matched with reference standard; quercetin

FRACTIONATION OF EXTRACTS AND THEIR CHROMATOGRAPHIC STUDIES

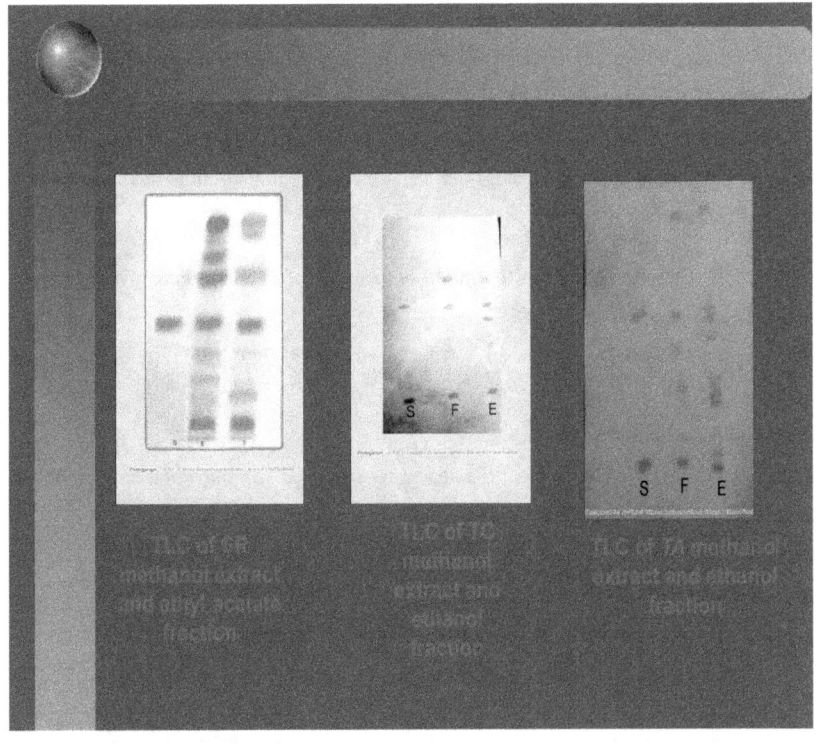

TLC of CR methanol extract and ethyl acetate fraction

TLC of TC methanol extract and ethanol fraction

TLC of TA methanol extract and ethanol fraction

5.4 HPLC OF FRACTIONS

HPLC is a separation technique in which mass-transfer occurs between stationary and mobile section (ICH guideline; **1996 and Devaliya R., Jain,U.K, 2009**). Fore the study Shimadzu HPLC System was used, which contains LC-10AT VP pumps, SCL-10A VP auto injector and Phenomenex Luna C18, 5 μm, (250 x 4.6 mm) column. and was used at ambient temperature.

5.4.1 HPLC Fingerprinting of Ethyl Acetate Fraction of *S. rebaudiana*

Chemicals and reagents employed:

Stevioside, >99.0% purity (Sigma), ethanol and acetonitrile(HPLC grade), phosphoric acid (analytical grade) were used.

Chromatographic conditions:

Mobile phase : HPLC grade acetonitrile and water was used as mobile phase, diluted with phosphoric acid. The solvent was filtered through 0.22μm-millipore filters.

Flow rate: 1.0 ml/min

Injection volume: 10 μl

Detector: UV at 265 nm using SPD – M10 AVP photodiode array detector.

Gradient elution

Time (Min.)	Acetonitrile (mL)	Water (mL)
0.01	20	80
25.0	25	75
35.0	35	65
40.0	40	60

Sample preparation for HPLC

100 mg of dry powdered sample (EAFSR) was dissolved in 50 ml of ethyl acetate, sonicated for 10 min volume made up to 100 ml with ethyl acetate and filtered .

Standard solutions:

In 10 ml volumetric flask 10 mg of stevioside dissolved in small amount of ethanol and finally volume made up with ethanol.

Procedure:

After adjusting instrument all filtered solutions were injected in volume of 10 µl according to protocol chromatograms were recorded. Retention times and peak area were noted. Quantity of stevioside within the sample was calculated.

Estimation:

The amount of stevioside present in the EAFSR in 10 µl was found to be 0.2793 µg **(Table 5.10)**. Therefore as per calculation 100 mg of ethyl acetate fraction would contain 2.793 mg of stevioside. The HPLC chromatogram of standard stevioside and ethyl acetate fraction of methanol extract were shown **(Figure 5.1 and 5.2)**.

Method validation

In order to validate the method of analysis to be used, validation protocol was developed for stevioside estimation, both reference standard were analyzed using various concentrations.

Preparation of stock solution:

The concentration of the main stock solutions for stevioside was calculated as mentioned below. Further six dilutions were made from the stock solution.

FRACTIONATION OF EXTRACTS AND THEIR CHROMATOGRAPHIC STUDIES

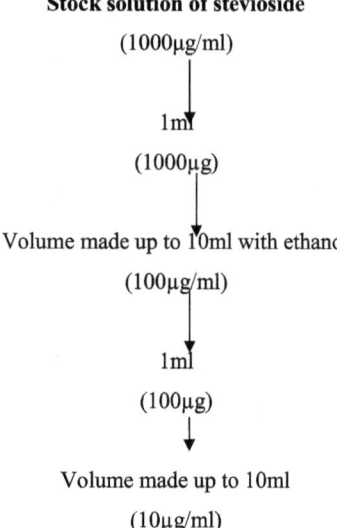

Flow chart 5.1 : Scheme of dilution for stevioside

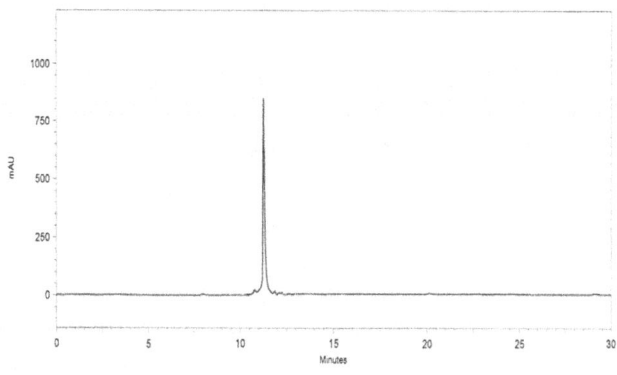

Figure 5.1 : HPLC chromatogram of standard stevioside

Retention time of standard stevioside

Peak	Retention time	Area	Height	% Area
1	11.54	392641	692682	100

Table 5.10 : Concentration and peak area of stevioside:

S.No.	Concentration (µg/mL)	Peak area
1	20	924102
2	40	1860456
3	80	3176948
4	160	62893282
5	320	11669508
6	640	22145620

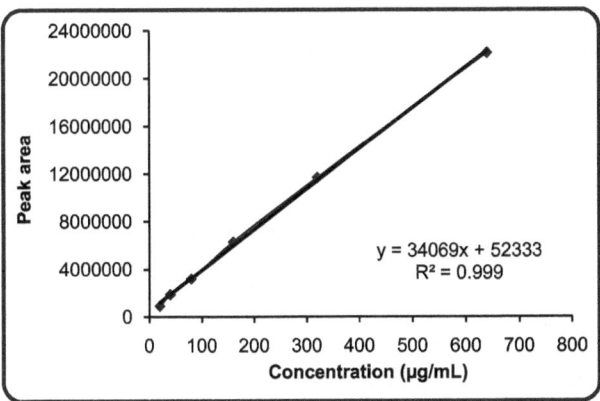

Graph 5.1 : Linearity graph between concentration vs. peak area of stevioside

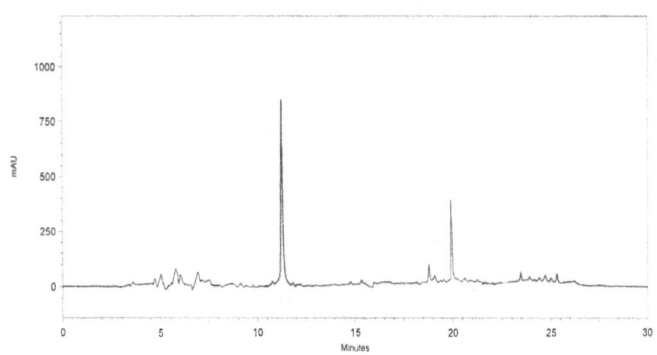

Peak	RT	Area	%Area	Height
1	11.54	53236	48.92	590584

Figure 5.2 : HPLC chromatogram of ethyl acetate fraction of *S. rebaudiana*

Table 5.11 : Estimation of stevioside by HPLC

Replicate	Sample area	stevioside (µg)
1	61753	0.2765
2	61906	0.2810
3	61889	0.2805
Average		0.2793

Procedure:

All the above six dilutions were injected and chromatograms were recorded. Linearity graphs with correlation co-efficient for stevioside was plotted respectively, using concentrations and the respective peak areas (Graph 5.1).

Limit of detection and limit of quantitation:

so as to estimate the limit of detection (LOD) and lower limit of quantitation (LOQ), the signal to noise quantitative relation (S/N) determined. LOD was thought of as 3:1 and LLOQ as 10:1. the boundaries were set at the concentration of lowest standardisation. The LOD and LLOQ were found to be 1.4 and 4.6 µg/mL.

FRACTIONATION OF EXTRACTS AND THEIR CHROMATOGRAPHIC STUDIES

Recovery studies:

The accuracy and exactness studied by standard addition technique in analyzed sample stevioside was added (0.4 µg, 0.6µg and 0.8 µg) sample, each level being repeated thrice. The recovered amount of drug and percentage recovery was calculated.

5.4.2 HPLC Fingerprinting of Ethanol Fraction of *T. cordifolia*

Chemicals and reagents employed:

Berberine >99.0% purity (Sigma), ethanol and acetonitrile(HPLC grade), phosphoric acid (analytical grade) were used.

Chromatographic conditions:

Mobile phase : HPLC grade acetonitrile and water (40:60) was used as mobile phase, diluted with phosphoric acid. The solvent was filtered through 0.22µm-millipore filters.

Flow rate: 1.0 ml/min

Injection volume: 10 µl

Detector: UV at 266 nm using SPD – M10 AVP photodiode array detector.

Gradient elution

Time (Min.)	Acetonitrile (mL)	Water (mL)
0.01	20	80
25.0	30	70
35.0	35	65
40.0	40	60

Sample preparation for HPLC

100 mg powdered sample (EFTC) of *T. cordifolia* was dissolved in 80 ml of ethanol after sonication made the volume to 100 ml with ethanol and filtered .

Preparation of Standard solutions

In 10 ml volumetric flask 10 mg of berberine dissolved in small amount of ethanol and finally volume made up with ethanol.

FRACTIONATION OF EXTRACTS AND THEIR CHROMATOGRAPHIC STUDIES

Procedure:

After adjusting instrument all filtered solutions were injected in volume of 10 µl according to protocol chromatograms were recorded. Retention times and peak area were noted. Quantity of berberine within the sample was calculated.

Method validation

In order to validate the method of analysis to be used, validation protocol was developed for berberine estimation, both reference standard were analyzed using various concentrations.

Preparation of stock solution:

The concentration of the main stock solutions for berberine was calculated as mentioned below. Further six dilutions were made from the stock solution.

Stock solution of berberine
(1000µg/ml)
↓ 1ml
(1000µg)
↓
Volume made up to 10ml with ethanol
(100µg/ml)
↓ 1ml
(100µg)
↓
Volume made up to 10ml
(10µg/ml)

Flow chart 5.2 : Scheme of dilution for berberine

Preparation of mobile Phase

To 40 part of acetonitrile and 60 part of water was mixed to get one liter of mobile phase after filtering sonicated for removal of gases

Procedure:

All the above six dilutions were injected and chromatograms were recorded. Linearity graphs with correlation co-efficient for berberine was plotted respectively, using concentrations and the respective peak areas (**Graph 5.2**).

Estimation:

The amount of berberine present in the EFTC in 10 µl was found to be 0.270 mg (**Table 5.12**). Therefore as per calculation 100 mg of ethanol fraction would contain 2.700 mg of stevioside. The HPLC chromatogram of standard berberine and ethanol fraction of methanol extract were shown (**Figure 5.3 and 5.4**).

Table 5.12 : Concentration and peak area of Berberine

S. No.	Concentration (µg/mL)	Peak area
1	20	1498012
2	40	2821424
3	80	5728468
4	160	11390753
5	320	22287245
6	640	44112785

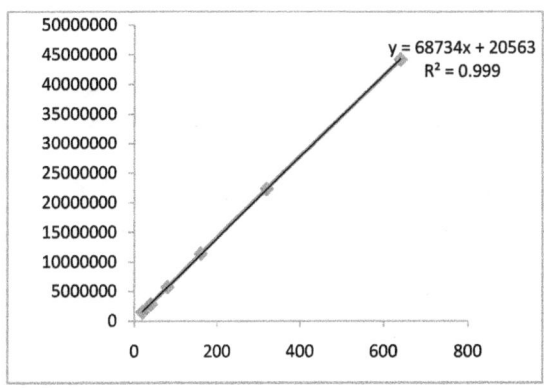

Graph 5.2 : Linearity graph between concentration vs. peak area of berberine

FRACTIONATION OF EXTRACTS AND THEIR CHROMATOGRAPHIC STUDIES

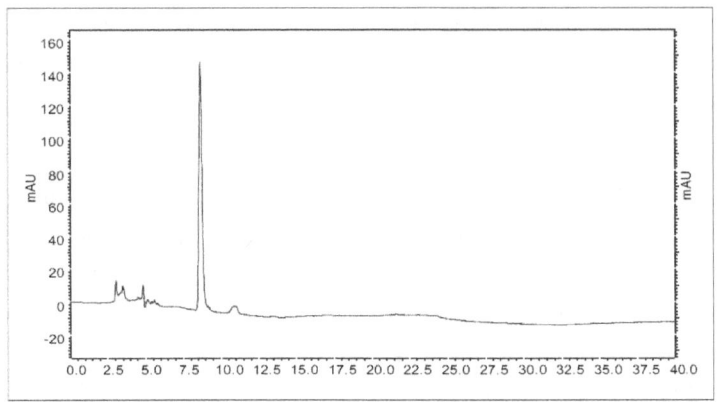

Peak	Retention time	Area	Height	% Area
1	8.35	1487012	629676	100

Figure 5.3 : HPLC chromatogram of standard Berberine

Table 5.13 : Estimation of berberine by HPLC

Replicate	Sample area	Berberine (µg)
1	1899012	0.0273
2	1868978	0.0268
3	1889567	0.0272
Average	645947±4329	0.027± 0.01

Mean ± SD, n=3

FRACTIONATION OF EXTRACTS AND THEIR CHROMATOGRAPHIC STUDIES

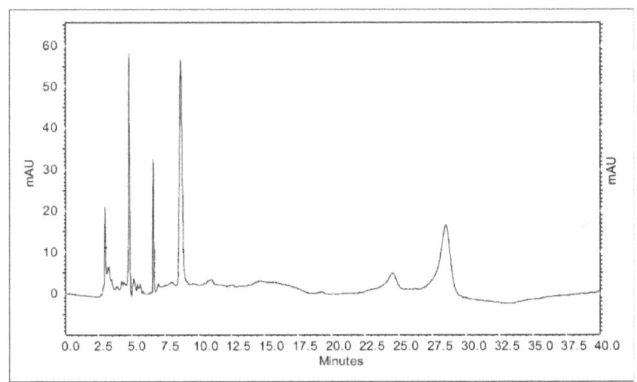

Peak	Retention time	Area	Height	% Area
1	8.34	1899012	269463	29.174%

Figure 5.4 : HPLC chromatogram of ethanol fraction of methanol extract of *T. cordifolia*

Calibration curve for berberine was obtained for the range of 20 to 640 µg/ml. for this calibration slope and intercept value was y=68734x2054. The method showed good linearity over the range of 20-640 µg/ml with (R^2) 0.999. Result was shown in the table-5.12 and 5.13 Figure 5.2.

Limit of detection and limit of quantitation:

So as to estimate the limit of detection (LOD) and lower limit of quantitation (LOQ), the signal to noise quantitative relation (S/N) determined. LOD was thought of as 3:1 and LLOQ as 10:1. the boundaries were set at the concentration of lowest standardisation. The LOD and LLOQ were found to be 1.4 and 4.6 µg/mL.

Recovery studies:

The accuracy and exactness studied by standard addition technique in analyzed sample berberine was added (0.4 µg, 0.6µg and 0.8 µg) sample, each level being repeated thrice. The recovered amount of drug and percentage recovery was calculated.

5.4.3 HPLC Fingerprinting of Ethanol fraction of T. aestivum (khan et al. 2015)

Chemicals and reagents employed:

quercetin, >99.0% purity (Sigma), HPLC grade of ethanol and acetonitrile, water, phosphoric acid in analytical grade were used.

Chromatographic system:

HPLC System (Shimadzu) comprising LC-10AT VP pumps, SCL-10A VP auto injector and Phenomenex Luna C18, 5 µm, (250 x 4.6 mm) column was used at ambient temperature.

Chromatographic conditions:

Mobile phase :

HPLC grade acetonitrile and 0.1%phosphoric acid (30:70)was used as mobile phase. The solvent was filtered through 0.22µm-millipore filters.

Flow rate : 1.0 ml/min

Injection volume : 10 µl

Detector : UV at 280nm using SPD–M10 AVP photodiode array detector.

Gradient elution

Time (Min.)	Acetonitrile (mL)	Water (mL)
0.01	15.0	85.0
25.0	25.0	75.0
30.0	35.0	65.0
35.0	45.0	55.0

Sample preparation for HPLC:

100 mg of dry powdered sample (ethanol fraction of methanol extract) of T. aestivum was dissolved in 80 ml of ethanol, sonicated for 10 min and diluted up to 100 ml with ethanol and filtered through 0.22µm millipore filters.

Standard solution:

Accurately weighed 10 mg of quercetin was placed into a 10 ml volumetric flask and dissolved in ethanol (stock solution).

Procedure:

All the above six dilutions were injected and chromatograms were recorded. Linearity graphs with correlation co-efficient for quercetin was plotted respectively, using concentrations and the respective peak areas **(Graph 5.3)**.

Estimation:

The amount of quercetin present in the ethanol fraction of methanol extract of TA fruits in 10 µl was found to be 0.6436 µg **(Table 5.15)**. Therefore 100 mg of ethanol fraction would contain 6.436 mg of quercetin. The HPLC chromatogram of standard quercetin and ethyl acetate fraction of methanol extract are shown **(Figure 5.5; 5.6)**.

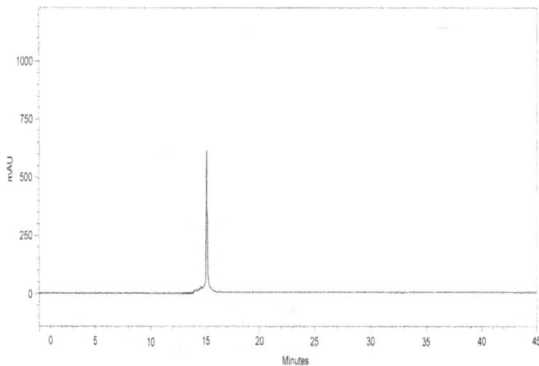

Retention time of standard quercetin

Peak	Retention time	Area	Height	% Area
1	**15.1**	1024488	**821680**	**100**

Figure5.5 : HPLC chromatogram of standard quercetin

FRACTIONATION OF EXTRACTS AND THEIR CHROMATOGRAPHIC STUDIES

Retention time of ethnol fraction of TA

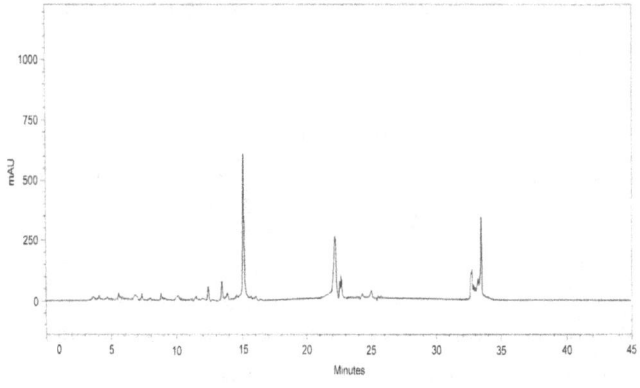

Peak	Retention time	Area	Height	% Area
1	15	62668.77	59435	37.65%

Figure 5.6 : HPLC chromatogram of ethyl acetate fraction of TA

Method validation:
In order to validate the method of analysis for estimation of quercetin, various concentrations were used.

Preparation of stock solution:
The concentration of the stock solutions for quercetin was calculated as mentioned below. Further six dilutions were made from the stock solution **(Flow chart 5.3)**.

FRACTIONATION OF EXTRACTS AND THEIR CHROMATOGRAPHIC STUDIES

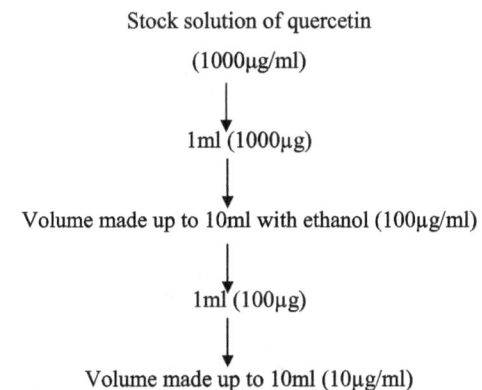

Flow chart 5.3 : Scheme of dilution quercetin

Procedure:

All the above six dilutions were injected and chromatograms were recorded. Linearity graphs with correlation co-efficient for quercetin was plotted, using concentrations on X-axis and the respective peak areas on Y-axis (**Graph 5.3**).

Table 5.14 : Concentration versus peak area of quercetin

S.No.	Concentration (µg/mL)	Peak area
1	20	1051422
2	40	1804218
3	80	3411426
4	160	6238450
5	320	11986316
6	640	23646035

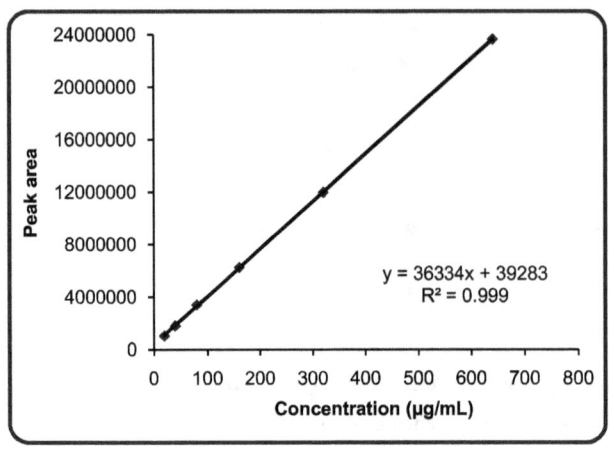

Graph 5.3: Linearity graph between concentrations vs. peak area of quercetin

Table 5.15 : Estimation of quercetin by HPLC

Replicate	Sample area	Quercetin (µg)
1	62627.59	0.6425
2	62427.76	0.6370
3	62950.97	0.6514
Average	**62668.77**	0.6436

Limit of detection and limit for quantification of quercetin:

In order to estimate the limit of detection (LOD) and lower limit of quantitation (LLOQ), the signal to noise ratio (S/N) was determined. LOD was considered as 3:1 and LLOQ as 10:1. The limits were set at the concentration of percentage recovery was calculated from recovered amount of drug.

FRACTIONATION OF EXTRACTS AND THEIR CHROMATOGRAPHIC STUDIES

Recovery studies:

The accuracy and exactness studied by standard addition technique in analyzed sample stevioside was added (0.4 µg, 0.6µg and 0.8 µg) sample, each level being repeated thrice. The recovered amount of drug and percentage recovery was calculated.

6. ANTIDIABETIC SCREENING OF FRACTIONS
6.1 ACUTE TOXICITY STUDIES

6.1.1 Selection of animals:

Albino rats were selectedand housed in well-ventilated rooms polypropylene cageswith proper availability of water and rat pellet feed.

6.1.2 Preparation of drug samples:

Fractions were prepared as 2% gum acacia suspensions. These were administrated through the oral route.

6.1.3 LD_{50} determination:

Fractions of extracts were subjected to Acute toxicity test as per the OECD guideline 423. Procedure was the same as that for crude extracts.

Table : 6.1 Acute toxicity study of fractions

S.No.	Fractions	LD_{50} Cut-off (mg/kg body weight)
1	BFSR	1000
2	EAFSR	1000
3	EFSR	1000
4	BFTC	1000
5	EAFMC	1000
6	EFTC	1000
7	BFTA	1000
8	EAFTA	1000
9	EFTA	1000

6.2 ANTIDIABETIC SCREENING

6.2.1 Scheme Of Antidiabetic Screening Models

Scheme discussed on earlier was followed.

Standard Drugs and Chemicals Used:

Kits for biochemical parameters such as Lipid profile, Total protein, Albumin, Creatinin and Urea, and Enzyme linked immunosorbent assay were purchased from Erba Diagnostics, Mannheim, Germany. Other chemicals were purchased from Sigma Aldrich Chemical and Qualigens.

Administration of samples:

Samples are administered orally in the form of 2% acacia suspension.

Statistical Analysis :

All the experimental knowledge for applied mathematics analysis, were conferred as mean±SEM. unidirectional analysis of variance (ANOVA) was applied by Dunnett's.

6.3 Acute Antidibetic Study Of Fractions

6.3.1 Effect of fractions on blood glucose in normal rats

The fractions of the extracts were subjected to determine the hypoglycemic activity at the dose levels (100, 200 and 400 mg/kg) in normal fasted rats without any prior history of drug treatment and the results are presented in **Table 6.2, Table 6.3** and **Table 6.4 and graph 6.1, 6.2, 6.3.**

ANTIDIABETIC EVALUATION OF PLANTS FRACTIONS

Table 6.2: Effect of SR fractions on BG in normal fasted rats.

S.No.	Treatment (mg/kg)	Blood glucose (mg/dl)			
		0 h (FBG)	2 h	4 h	6 h
1.	NC	86.6±2.48	86.80±1.65	85.95±2.51	86.00±3.02
2.	BFSR$_{50}$	86.12 ± 1.05	89.68±2.62	88.44±1.86	87.06±1.58
3.	BFSR$_{100}$	88.60 ± 2.20	89.31±2.22	90.78±2.24	88.66±1.72
4.	BFSR$_{200}$	85.00± 2.46	84.20±1.86	85.00±2.32	86.77±1.94
5.	EAFSR$_{50}$	85.2±3.12	83.4±1.78	82.8±1.80	83.0±2.65
6.	EAFSR$_{100}$	85.4±2.78	82.8±3.00	78.8±2.64 $^{a\ b}$	76.8±2.84 $^{a\ b}$
7.	EAFSR$_{200}$	83.6±3.13	80.2±2.65	75.5±1.87 $^{a\ b}$	73.8±2.83 $^{a\ b}$
8.	EFSR$_{50}$	86.00±1.09	87.30±2.56	89.24±1.90	89.70±2.05
9.	EFSR$_{100}$	88.70±2.82	85.53±1.96	87.00±2.42	87.10±2.62
10	EFSR$_{200}$	85.30±1.66	85.19±1.28	84.10±2.56	83.12±1.68
11.	GLB	88.25±2.20	86.10±2.22	76.54±2.92 $^{a\ b}$	68.44±2.45 $^{a\ b}$

Table 6.3: Effect of TC fractions on BG in normal fasted rats.

S.No.	Treatment (mg/kg)	0 h (FBG)	2 h	4 h	6 h
1	NC	87.8±2.12	87.5±1.96	87.34±2.82	87.62±2.24
2	BFTC$_{50}$	85.8±1.89	83.6±3.00	83.8±2.56	84.8±2.00
3	BFTC$_{100}$	84.2±2.87	84.6±2.45	82.2±2.68	83.8±2.42
4	BFTC$_{200}$	83.8±2.56	81.2±2.35	81.6±2.88	82.8±3.01
5	EAFTC$_{50}$	85.12±3.01	85.6±1.67	86.96±2.68	85.02±2.90
6	EAFTC$_{100}$	86.12±1.36	89.68±2.18	88.44±2.35	87.06±1.83
7	EAFTC$_{200}$	88.6±2.32	89.31±3.35	90.78±1.88	88.66±1.55
8	EFTC$_{50}$	85.21±2.4	84.21±3.23	85.44±1.50	86.77±1.12
9	EFTC$_{100}$	90.47±4.16	87.43±2.36	81.20±2.02 $^{a\ b}$	72.40±1.32 $^{a\ b}$
10	EFTC$_{200}$	85.20±1.49	84.29±1.58	78.22±2.31$^{a\ b}$	70.33±2.72 $^{a\ b}$
11	GLB	86.40±1.28	83.94±3.02	74.10±2.32 $^{a\ b}$	65.54±2.86 $^{a\ b}$

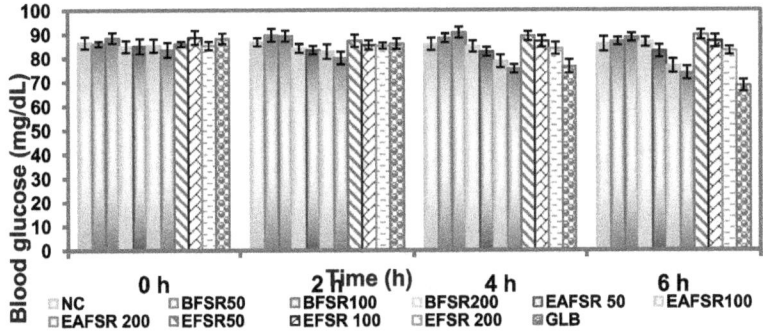

Graph 6.1: Effect of SR fractions on BG in normal fasted rats.

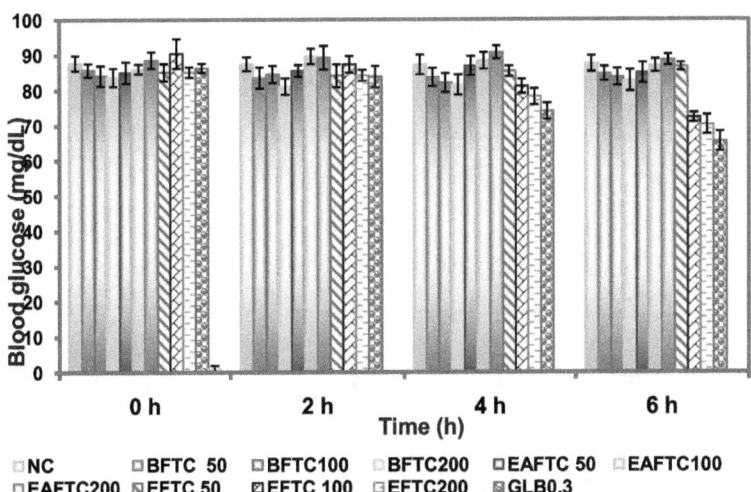

Graph 6.2: Effect of TC fractions on BG in normal fasted rats.

Table 6.4: Effects of TA fractions in fasted normal rats.

ANTIDIABETIC EVALUATION OF PLANTS FRACTIONS

S.No.	Treatment (mg/kg)	Blood glucose (mg/dl)			
		0 h (FBG)	2 h	4 h	6 h
1.	NC	86.26±1.9	86.08±2.54	86.45±2.64	86.42±2.14
2.	$BFTA_{50}$	85.28±3.02	86.00±2.42	85.86±2.30	85.25±1.80
3.	$BFTA_{100}$	87.74±2.86	88.10±3.14	88.00±1.42	88.250±3.15
4.	$BFTA_{200}$	86.50±3.02	86.46±3.02	86.78± 3.01	86.18±2.32
5.	$EAFTA_{50}$	88.03±2.32	84.55±1.55	85.30±1.50	86.65±2.13
6.	$EAFTA_{100}$	87.62±3.32	86.43±2.06	88.00±2.52	87.10±1.12
7.	$EAFTA_{200}$	86.20±3.00	85.60±1.96	86.28±2.62	86.00±2.22
8.	$EFTA_{50}$	88.80±1.96	87.96±2.30	88.40±3.12	88.15±2.08
9.	$EFTA_{100}$	86.00±2.34	86.20±1.42	85.73±2.02	85.90±1.84
10	$EFTA_{200}$	87.30±1.60	85.60±1.76	86.00±2.66	86.80±2.32
11.	GLB	85.340±2.69	84.46±2.72	74.04±2.80 $^{a\,b}$	64.24±2.26 $^{a\,b}$

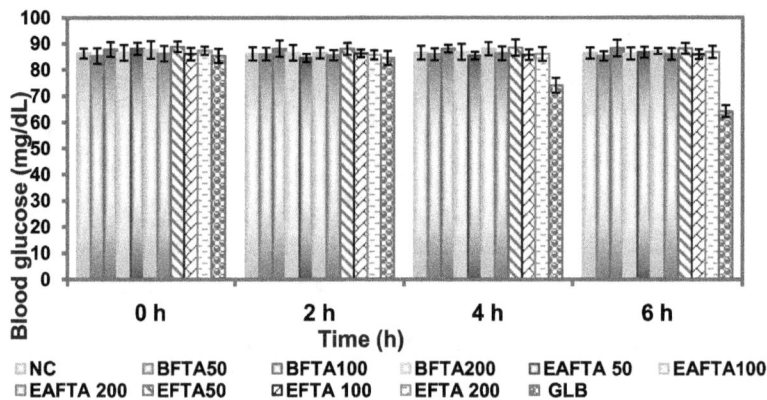

Graph 6.3 : Effect of TA fractions on BG in normal fasted rats.

6.3.2 Effect of of fractions on OGTT in normal rats

Administered 1.0 g/kg body wt of glucose, orally to overnight fasted animals. Standard group received glibenclamide, treated groups received different fractions, control groups received only vehicle, before the administration of glucose. B. G was estimated from 30 min to 2h.

Table : 6.5 Effect of SR fractions on OGTT in normal fasted rats.

S.No.	Treatment (mg/kg)	Blood glucose concentration(mg/dl)			
		0h(FBG)	1/2h	1h	2h
1	NC+ Glucose	87.42±4.32	165.50±4.16	128.08±3.48	91.20±2.12
2	$BFSR_{50}$+ Glucose	86.28±2.84	154.24±5.62	136.32 ± 4.70	112.45± 4.36
3	$BFSR_{100}$+ Glucose	88.48± 5.60	168.62±7.12	145.81 ± 2.96	116.20± 5.20
4	$BFSR_{200}$+ Glucose	87.22± 4.48	158.60± 6.06	142.26 ±5.92	100.54 ± 5.10
5	$EAFSR_{50}$+ Glucose	87.32±3.88	132.60±6.80 [a]	104.54 ± 5.00	98.46± 3.90
6	$EAFSR_{100}$+ Glucose	88.54± 3.04	124.80± 4.46 [a]	98.22 ± 5.60	94.72 ± 3.08
7	$EAFSR_{200}$+ Glucose	85.46± 3.62	120.32± 4.07 [a]	94.14± 3.10	88.52 ± 5.38
8	$EFSR_{50}$+ Glucose	85.62±2.60	160.62±4.28	144.32 ± 4.70	112.20± 4.04
9	$EFSR_{100}$+ Glucose	86.80± 3.18	158.00± 7.20	137.80 ± 6.60	108.20± 5.20
10	$EFSR_{200}$+ Glucose	88.80± 4.76	160.60± 4.76	136.42 ± 6.72	107.40 ± 6.10
11	GLB+ Glucose	86.24±4.10	110.40±4.12 [a]	92.10 ± 4.98	88.50±5.10

Table 6.6: Effect of TC fractions on OGTT in normal fasted rats.

S. No.	Treatment(mg/kg)	Blood glucose concentration(mg/dl)			
		0h(FBG)	1/2h	1h	2h
1	NC+ Glucose	86.4±1.92	168.36±6.24	120.51±3.98	108.1±3.05
2	BFTC$_{50}$+ Glucose	83.28±6.04	163.34 ± 4.80	154.36 ±6.54	106.26± 5.43
3	BFTC$_{100}$+ Glucose	88.45± 5.42	170.53± 3.24	156.00 ± 6.24	95.42± 6.18
4	BFTC$_{200}$+ Glucose	85.67± 6.18	167.46± 4.48	158.40 ± 7.06	97.29 ± 4.86
5	EAFTC$_{50}$+ Glucose	85.24± 3.12	166.5 ± 6.15	156.20 ± 7.23	102.24± 5.20
6	EAFTC$_{100}$+ Glucose	86.82±4.62	162.56 ± 4.58	154.46 ± 6.54	93.06 ± 5.64
7	EAFTC$_{200}$+ Glucose	85.64±4.20	162.32 ± 6.00	152.80 ± 5.02	100.45± 6.42
8	EFTC$_{50}$+ Glucose	87.42±4.80	121.40± 3.12 [a]	118.14 ± 4.10	89.48± 4.62
9	EFTC$_{100}$+ Glucose	90.12± 5.84	120.46 ± 5.04	108.64± 4.45 [a]	92.20± 3.12
10	EFTC$_{200}$+ Glucose	88.32±5.36	116.65 ± 4.38	102.60± 5.04 [a]	89.40 ± 3.10
11	GLB+ Glucose	85.2±3.56	106.2±6.23 [a]	95.4 ± 4.02	86.1±3.62

ANTIDIABETIC EVALUATION OF PLANTS FRACTIONS

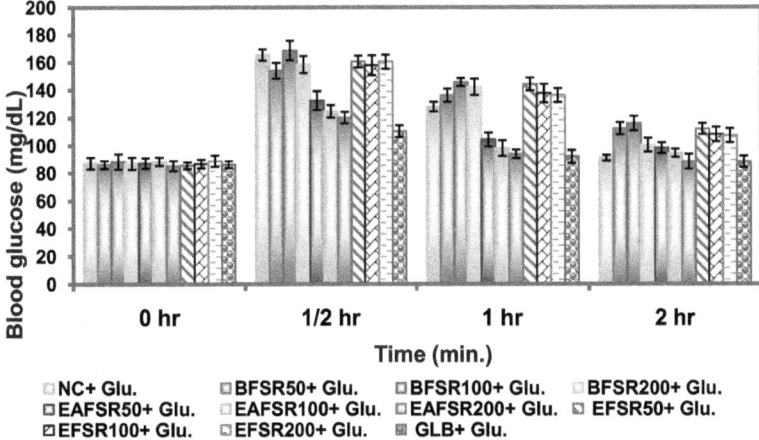

Graph 6.4: Effect of SR fractions on OGTT in normal fasted rats.

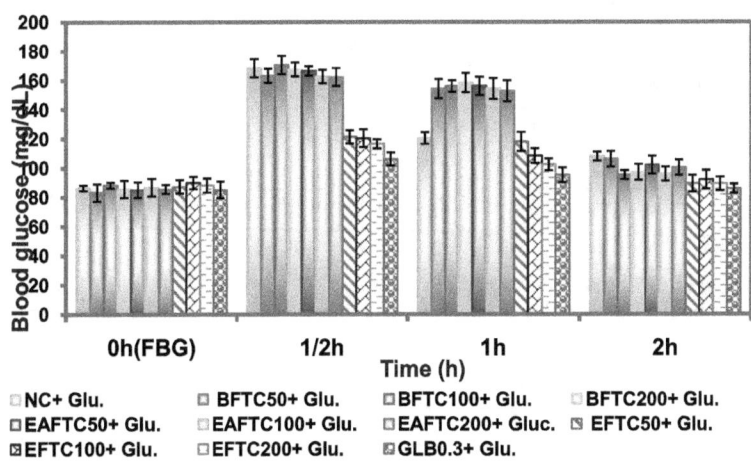

Graph 6.4: Graph 6.5: Effect of TC fractions on OGTT in normal fasted rats.

Table 6.7: Effect of fractions of TA on OGTT in normal fasted rats.

S.No.	Treatment (mg/kg)	Blood glucose concentration(mg/dl)			
		0h(FBG)	1/2h	1h	2h
1	NC+ Glucose	87.28±2.92	160.5±4.25	92.6±5.64	90.68±3.75
2	$BFTA_{50}$+ Glucose	86.62±4.60	164.64±4.38	146.32 ± 5.70	99.20± 4.04
3	$BFTA_{100}$+ Glucose	87.80± 5.18	166.00± 8.20	139.80 ± 3.60	96.20± 5.20
4	$BFTA_{200}$+ Glucose	86.80± 3.76	165.60± 5.76	138.42 ± 7.72	97.40 ± 6.10
5	$EAFTA_{50}$+ Glucose	88.00±3.10	152.30± 9.12	93.40 ± 6.48	88.46± 3.42
6	$EAFTA_{100}$+ Glucose	86.60± 2.68	154.00± 3.66	92.20 ± 6.30	86.20 ± 2.80
7	$EAFTA_{200}$+ Glucose	83.30± 4.82	149.60± 7.60	88.60± 4.14	87.40 ± 7.16
8	$EFTA_{50}$+ Glucose	84.20±6.23	121.62± 3.45 [a]	134.76 ± 5.54	92.44± 8.12
9	$EFTA_{100}$+ Glucose	81.06± 5.88	116.80± 5.00 [a]	132.60 ± 5.16	95.20± 9.38
10	$EFTA_{100}$+ Glucose	90.68± 5.90	111.20± 4.97 [a]	132.40 ± 8.28	96.24 ± 8.10
11	GLB+ Glucose	88.8±3.12	101.2±5.10 [a]	90.4 ± 3.98	87.0±4.60

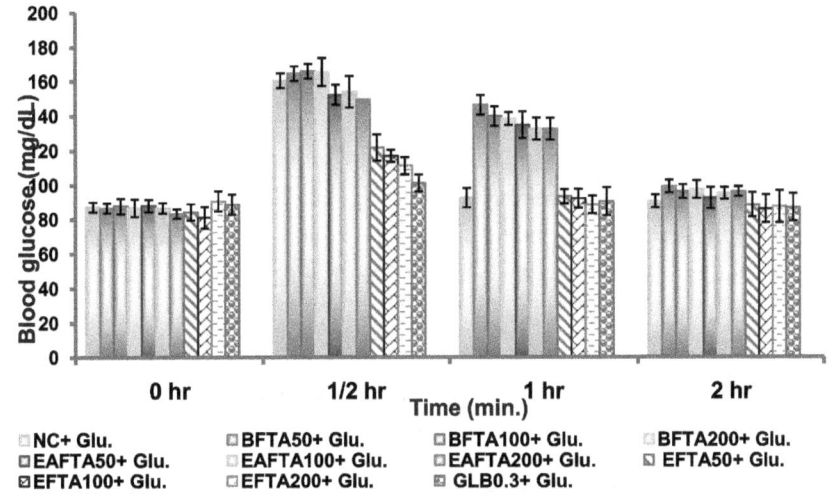

Graph 6.6 : Effect of TA fractions on OGTT in normal fasted rats.

ANTIDIABETIC EVALUATION OF PLANTS FRACTIONS

6.3.3 Effect of fractions on BG in streptozotocin induced diabetic rats – acute antidiabetic activity

6.3.3.1 Induction of diabetes

Due to instability of STZ in aqueous media, before use it's solution is prepared in citrate buffer (pH 4.5), intraperitoneally injected (45 mg/kg) in rats then allowed a rest period of 2 days with free access of food and water **(Brosky and Logothelopoulos, 1969)**. The rats have FBG more than 250 mg/dl were selected for the study.

6.3.3.2 BG estimation

FBG of over night fasted NC DC SC and fraction treated group of animals was done. Blood glucose estimated at 2, 4 and 6h. after appropriate treatments

Table 6.8 : Effect of SR fractions on BG level in streptozotocin induced diabetic rats.

S.No.	Treatment (mg/kg)	Blood glucose (mg/dl)			
		0 h(FBG)	2 h	4 h	6 h
1.	DC	272.08±6.80	272.60±8.46	273.20±9.40	272.24±10.52
2.	$BFSR_{50}$	280.30±7.28	281.12±8.02	282.10±10.02	320.20 ±6.86
3.	$BFSR_{100}$	276.52±4.80	275.80±5.30	273.00±7.24	275.48±9.84
4.	$BFSR_{200}$	286.60±10.28	286.30±6.20	284.40±8.08	285.02±10.40
5.	$EAFSR_{50}$	278.84±6.48	270.40±9.07	236.38±8.51 [a,b]	203.42±7.42 [a,b]
6.	$EAFSR_{100}$	282.24±11.64	252.74±8.28 [a,b]	230.20±9.42 [a,b]	195.52±10.70 [a,b]
7.	$EAFSR_{200}$	288.68±9.12	264.62±7.90 [a,b]	240.46±6.20 [a,b]	190.10±8.46 [a,b]
8.	$EFSR_{50}$	270.46±8.82	271.34±7.64	269.32±8.90	269.80±9.12
9.	$EFSR_{100}$	278.68±5.82	280.40±9.48	279.86±10.25	278.28±10.62
10.	$EFSR_{200}$	272.00±11.32	273.60±9.46	271.92±10.46	271.50±8.80
11.	GLB	288.00±6.86	246.30±6.48 [a,b]	208.26± 7.66 [a,b]	189.20± 5.28 [a,b]

Table 6.9: Effect of TC fractions on BG level in s induced diabetic rats.

S.No.	Treatment (mg/kg)	Blood glucose (mg/dl)			
		0 h(FBG)	2 h	4 h	6 h
1.	DC	286.20±5.10	287.32±6.60	287.60±8.12	287.84±6.40
2.	$BFTC_{50}$	292.30±8.20	292.65±7.18	291.90±10.00	292.00±7.62
3.	$BFTC_{100}$	290.24±8.24	291.82±7.80	292.00±11.02	291.40±6.40
4.	$BFTC_{200}$	289.62±4.90	289.68±6.32	289.50±9.10	289.26±7.08
5.	$EAFTC_{50}$	298.44±7.10	298.25±6.50	299.16±8.62	298.56±9.28
6.	$EAFTC_{100}$	290.24±8.24	291.82±7.80	292.00±9.10	291.40±6.40
7.	$EAFTC_{200}$	308.20±8.40	308.82±9.02	307.46±10.32	308.74±9.06
8.	$EFTC_{50}$	298.36±9.18	270.62±8.98 ^{ab}	236.4±7.88 ^{ab}	212.42±7.42 ^{ab}
9.	$EFTC_{100}$	302.40±10.26	268.62±9.18 ^{ab}	226.08±8.72 ^{ab}	207.35±8.42 ^{ab}
10.	$EFTC_{200}$	300.45±8.20	262.02±7.20 ^{ab}	221.42±5.16 ^{ab}	200.10±8.46 ^{ab}
11.	GLB	290.00±6.10	246.30±5.85 ^{ab}	202.12±6.40 ^{ab}	198.20±6.20 ^{ab}

ANTIDIABETIC EVALUATION OF PLANTS FRACTIONS

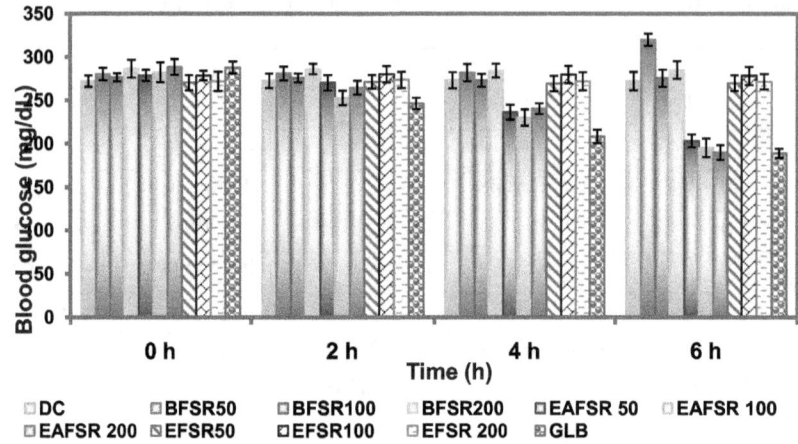

Graph 6.7 Effect of SR fractions on BG level in s induced diabetic rats.

Table 6.10: Effect of TA fractions on BG level in STZ induced diabetic rats.

S.No.	Treatment (mg/kg)	Blood glucose (mg/dl)			
		0 h (FBG)	2 h	4 h	6 h
1.	DC	281.08±10.02	284.10±9.56	280.21±9.84	282.24±11.00
2.	BFTA$_{50}$	284.00±10.45	285.80±10.20	285.10± 10.40	282.00± 8.46
3.	BFTA$_{100}$	283.20±11.38	282.40±11.30	284.40± 9.86	285.20 ± 9.58
4.	BFTA$_{200}$	276.45±8.72	276.2± 10.00	276.20± 9.84	275.60 ± 8.02
5.	EAFTA$_{50}$	276.20±9.60	274.52±9.08	274.00± 10.05	275.40 ± 10.80
6.	EAFTA$_{100}$	268.64±10.08	268.20± 10.94	266.76±8.90	268.86 ± 10.30
7.	EAFTA$_{200}$	272.84±11.40	271.00±8.33	274.05± 10.00	274.80 ± 10.70
8.	EFTA$_{50}$	288.00±7.84	284.20±9.80	272.20± 9.34	234.46* ± 9.50
9.	EFTA$_{100}$	280.54±11.02	258.80± 9.10 ^{ab}	224.50± 8.16 ^{ab}	217.71±7.86 ^{ab}
10.	EFTA$_{200}$	289.80±9.48	260.80±10.60 ^{ab}	243.20 ± 9.82 ^{ab}	218.22±4.04 ^{ab}
11.	GLB$_{0.3}$	288.00±7.02	248.25±6.20 ^{ab}	211.40± 5.72 ^{ab}	202.80± 8.24 ^{ab}

ANTIDIABETIC EVALUATION OF PLANTS FRACTIONS

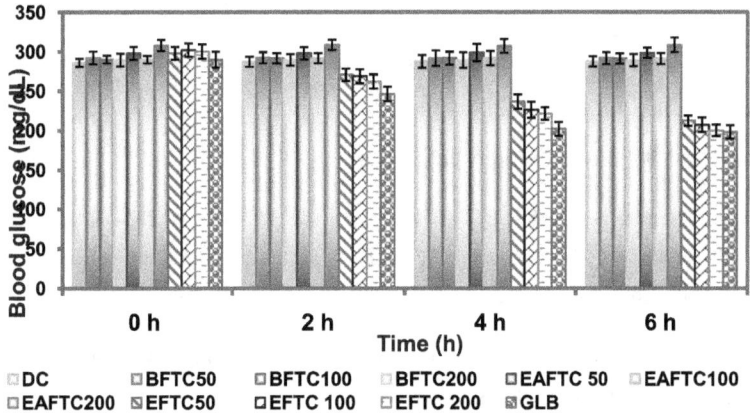

Graph 6.8: Effect of TC fractions on BG level in STZ induced diabetic rats

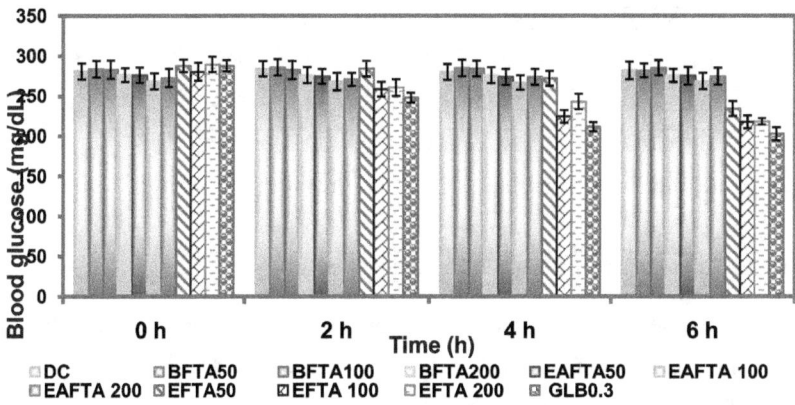

Graph 6.9: Effect of TA fractions on blood glucose level in STZ induced diabetic rats

ANTIDIABETIC EVALUATION OF PLANTS FRACTIONS

6.4 Four Weeks Treatment Of Fractions In STZ Induced Diabetic Rats

As per the result of acute study EAFSR, EFTC and EFTA were selected for further study.

6.4.1 Effect on BG in STZ induced diabetic rats

Each fractions i.e EAFSR, EFTC and EFTA was administered 28days daily at the dose of 100 mg/kg and Glibenclamide 0.30 mg/kg, p.o. as a standard drug orally in STZ-induced diabetic rats and determined the BG. (**Table 6.11; Graph 6.10**).

Table 6.11: Effects of four weeks administration of different fractions on blood glucose level in streptozotocin induced diabetic rats.

S. No.	Treatment	BG(mg/dl)	
		Before Treatment	After Treatment
1.	Normal control	82.62±4.00	81.24±4.30
2.	Diabetic control	282.24±6.36	300.45±6.20**
3.	EAFSR100	298.20±6.34	134.50±4.50*
4.	EFTC100	296.64±6.08	122.51±5.22*
5.	EFTA100	288.40±7.08	128.62±6.10*
6.	GLB	290.30±6.14	126.20±4.12*

6.4.2 Effect on Lipid Profile in STZ induced diabetic rats

After twenty eight days of treatment, macromolecule profile was calculated, in line with the directions of kits. LDL and VLDL were calculated by formula of Friedwald et al.,1972 . VLDL cholesterol = Triglycerides/5 and LDL = Total cholesterol − (VLDL+HDL cholesterol). The obtained lipid profile results were expressed in mg/dl. (**Table 6.12; Graph 6.11**).

Table 6.12 : Effect of four weeks treatment of EAFSR, EFTC and EFTA on lipid profile in STZ-induced diabetic rats.

S.No	Treatment (mg/kg)	Cholesterol (mg/dl)	HDL (mg/dl)	LDL (mg/dl)	VLDL (mg/dl)	TG (mg/dl)
1.	NC	84.12±4.80	40.28±2.30	26.32± 3.10	17.52±1.6*	87.62±7.26
2.	DC	146.82±1.40**	25.0±1.86**	92.14±7.64**	29.68±1.4**	148.42±5.06**
3.	EAFSR	123.06±3.08*	42.46±3.04*	50.25±3.10*	30.35±1.8*	31.2±5.13*
4.	EFTC	114.44±3.96*	34.00±2.30*	56.30±4.20*	24.14±1.9*	120.68±5.16*
5.	EFTA	104.46±5.18*	34.98±2.10*	49.06±3.82*	20.42±1.1	102.12±4.38*
6.	GLB	112.32±6.52*	39.05±1.24*	46.86±2.18*	26.41±2.1*	132.06±4.44*

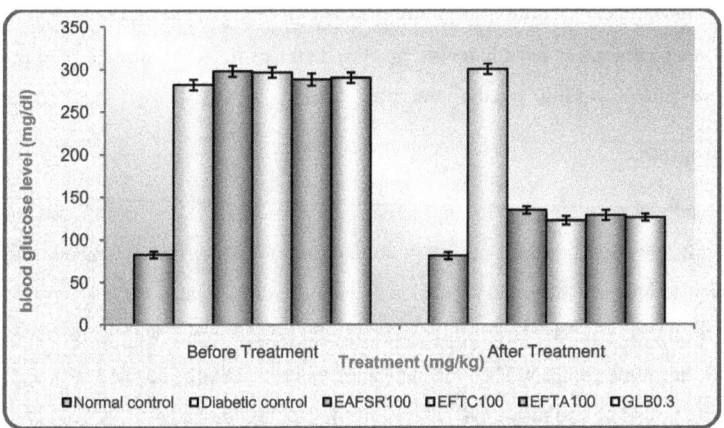

Graph 6.10: Effects of four weeks administration of fractions on BG level in STZ induced diabetic rats.

ANTIDIABETIC EVALUATION OF PLANTS FRACTIONS

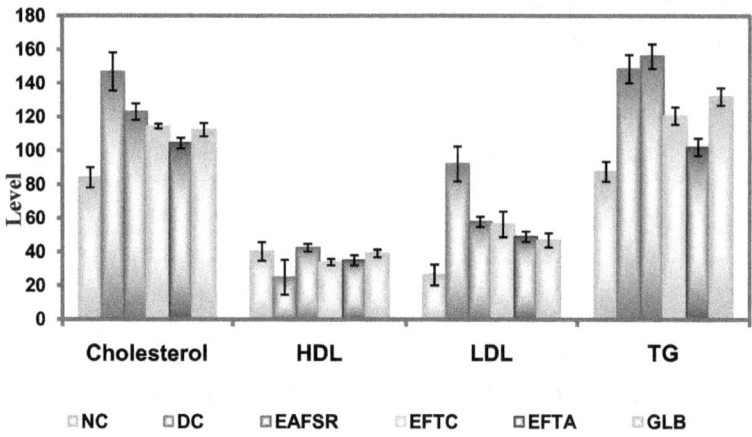

Graph 6.11: Effect on lipid profile in STZ-induced diabetic rats

6.4.3 Effect on biochemical parameter as Insulin, Total protein, Albumin, Creatinin and Urea in streptozotocin induced diabetic rats

Estimation of insulin:

The insulin assay done by using Mercodia insulin ELISA kits from Uppsala, Sweden. Estimation is based on the Principle of solid phase two-site enzyme immunoassay, direct sandwich technique where two monoclonal antibodies are directed against separate antigenic determinants(Gerich and Smith, 2003). insulin intreact with peroxidase-conjugated anti-insulin antibodies. Then bound conjugate was estimated reaction with 3, 3, 5, 5'-tetramethylbenzidine and measured . at 450 nm spectrophotometrically.

Procedure:

Before proceeding with the assay, all reagents, serum references and control were brought to room temperature (22-25°C).

The microplate wells were formatted and 50µl of the appropriate calibrators, controls and samples were pipetted into assigned wells. 100 µl of the enzyme labeled antibodies were added to each well. After 20-30 sec mix and covered with a plastic wrap and incubated for 120 minutes at room temperature (22-25OC). discarded the contents washed with buffer and decanted. 100µl of operating substrate solution was added to all wells, incubated at room temperature for 15 minutes and mixed with 50 µl of stock solution. Within 30 minutes absorbance were taken at 450nm in a microplate reader.

Estimation of protein

Serum protein was resolute in keeping with the strategy of **Reinhold(1980)**. The amide bonds of supermolecule produce blue-violet colour on reacting with copper II ions in alkaline media. Tartarate was added as a device while Iodide was employed to forestall auto-reduction of the alkalic copper complex, measured colour at 520- 560nm.

Estimation of Albumin

On binding with Bromocresol green, Albumin inflicting a shift in absorbance at pH 4.2, when measured photometrically between 580-630 nm with maximum absorbance at 625nm **(Tietz,1986)**. Albumin Reagent contains Bromocresol green, Sodium Azide, Succinate Buffer (pH 4.2 ± 0.1 at 25^0 C) and Surfactant. Albumin Standard contains 3.6g/dl

Estimation of Urea:

Done according to **Tiffany et al ,1972**. Urea. Sample and Standard mixed well with reagent (α – Ketoglutarate, NADH, Urease, GLDH, ADP, Tris Buffer pH 7.9 , fillers along with stabillizers).

It involve following reactions:

$$Urea + H_2O \xrightarrow{Urease} 2NH_3 + CO_2$$

$$NH_3 + \alpha\text{-KG} + NADH \xrightarrow{GLDH} Glutamate + NAD$$

α - KG: α - Ketoglutarate

GLDH: Glutamate dehydrogenase

Urea Reagent contains. Standard contains 50 mg /dl (23.4 mg /dl) of Urea.

$$\text{Urea (mg/dl)} = \frac{\Delta A \text{ of test}}{\Delta A \text{ of standard}} \times \text{Concentration of Standard (mg/d)}$$

Where $\Delta A = A_1 - A_2$, is rate of decrease in absorbance mesured at 340 nm.

Table 6.13: Effect on Insulin, Total protein, Albumin and Urea in STZ-induced diabetic rats

S. No.	Treatment (mg/kg)	Insulin	Total protein	Albumin	Urea
1.	NC	13.10±0.54	9.64±0.62	3.74±0.18	32.80±0.52
2.	DC	5.25±1.32**	8.07±0.26**	2.60±0.20**	70.60±0.78**
3.	EAFSR	9.50±0.38*	8.65±0.28**	2.78±0.54**	38.50±0.44*
4.	EFTC	10.42±2.16*	9.80±1.20*	3.25±0.12*	36.80±1.80*
5.	EFTA	10.92±1.76*	10.05±0.36*	3.35±0.14*	35.83±0.52*
6.	GLB	11.10±1.42*	10.12±0.68*	3.52±0.10*	32.90±0.48*

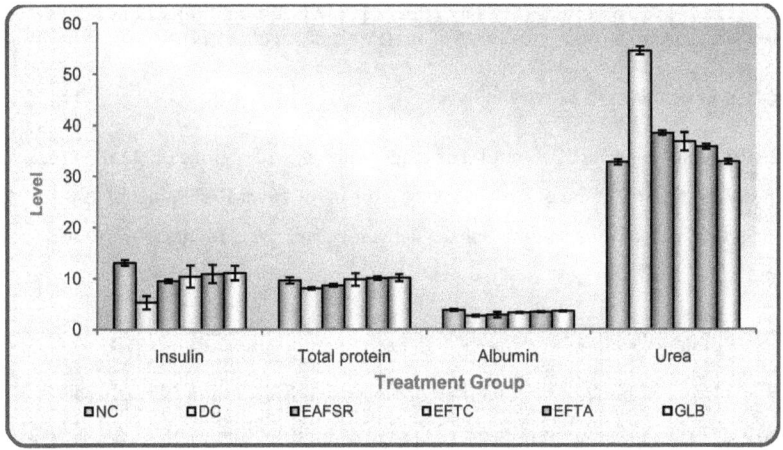

Graph 6.12 Effect on Insulin, Total protein, Albumin and Urea in STZ-induced diabetic rats

6.4.4 Effect on activity of on glucose-6-phosphatase, hexokinase and glycogen in STZ-induced diabetic rats

Hexokinase play important role in glucose metabolism. It causes impaired glucose oxidation glycolysis resulting hyperglycemia. Glucose-6-phosphatase and fructose-1,6-bisphosphatase, are the regulatory enzymes in gluconeogenic pathway. glucose-6-phosphatase incresed during fasting and at low glucose levels (**Schaftingen and Gerin 2002**). .

Estimation of glucose–6–phosphatase activities in liver

The tissue samples were homogenized in 250 mM ice-cold sucrose solution . For the reaction, (100 mM pH 6.5) and 0.1 ml of liver homogenate were added and thoroughly mixed. The reaction mixtures which contains 0.1 ml of sucrose/EDTA buffer (0.25 M / 0.001 M, sucrose/EDTA solution), 0.1 ml of 100 mM glucose-6-phosphate, 0.1 ml of imidazole buffer incubated at 37°C for 15 min. added 2 ml of Ascorbate (3%w/v) and centrifuged at 3,000 rpm for 10 min. separated the supernatant. After 0.5 ml of ammonium molybdate (1% w/v) and 1 ml of sodium citrate (2% w/v) absorbance was measured with spectrophotometrically at 700 nm**(Baginsky et al., 1974)**..

Estimation of hexokinase activity in liver:

To liver tissue homogenate 22.8 ml of Tris magnesium chloride buffer (200 mM Tris and 20 mM $MgCl_2$, pH 8) , 0.5 ml of 0.67 M glucose, 0.1 ml of 16 mM ATP, 0.1 ml of 6.8 mM NAD and 0.01 ml of gluose-6-phosphate dehydrogenase. at 340 nm absorbance was measured.

Estimation of Glycogen by chemical method:

Centrifuged liver and skeleton muscles after homogenized with warm 80% ethanol for 20 min at 10,000 rpm. After drying 5 ml of DW and 6 ml of perchloric acid was added. Extracted for 20 min. at 4°C further centrifuged for 15 min at 10,000 rpm made up the volume of supernatant 1 ml with DW. Added 4 ml of anthrone reagent, incubated at for 10 min. The absorbances measured at 630 nm. **(Maiti et al., 2004)**.

Table :6.14 Effect of fractions on enzymes in streptozotocin-induced diabetic rats

S.No.	Treatment (mg/kg)	Enzyme level		Glycogen content estimation (mg /g of tissue)	
		Glucose-6phosphatase	Hexokinase	Liver Glycogen	Muscles Glycogen
1.	NC	0.182±0.004	0.144±0.002	31.4±2.1	5.6±0.3
2.	DC	0.324±0.008**	0.092±0.03**	19.2±0.8**	3.2±0.3**
3.	EAFSR	0.165±0.005*	0.124±0.05*	25.8±1.3*	4.4±0.4*
4.	EFTC	0.174±0.006*	0.132±0.008*	26.1±1.4*	4.8±0.3*
5.	EFTA	0.181±0.004*	0.138±0.007*	27.6±1.5*	5.1±0.2*
6.	GLB	0.176±0.003*	0.148±0.004*	28.1±1.4*	5.8±0.3*

6.4.5 Effect on SGOT and SGPT:

In diabetic animals the change in the levels of serum enzymes are directly related to changes in the metabolism in which the enzyme is involved the metabolism in which the enzyme is involved.

SGPT estimated as the strategy of **Bradley et al;1972**. SGPT Reagent(L-alanine, NADH,LDH, 2-Oxoglutarate, 7.5 pH Buffer, non- reactive fillers and stabilizers) was mixed with sample. The mean absorbance change per min for every reading was determined. SGOT Reagent (2-Oxoglutarate, L-Aspartate, MDH, LDH, NADH,EDTA Buffer pH 7.8±0.1 at 25°C, non- reactive fillers and stabilizers) was mixed with sample and the reactants were kept at room temp for 10min. and absorbance was read at 546nm(**Bergmeyer et al;1974**).

Table 6.15: Effect on SGOT,SGPT in streptozotocin-induced diabetic rats

S.No.	Treatment (mg/kg)	SGOT	SGPT
1.	Normal control	76.5±4.2	57.8±3.6
2.	Diabetic control	223.6±7.2**	138.2±7.2**
3.	EAFAM	124.2±6.2*	92.4±6.5*
4.	EAFMC	116.8±7.1*	81.2±5.0*
5.	EFTC	82.5±5.2*	79.4±4.8*
6.	GLB (0.3mg)	98.2±5.6*	81.4±5.2*

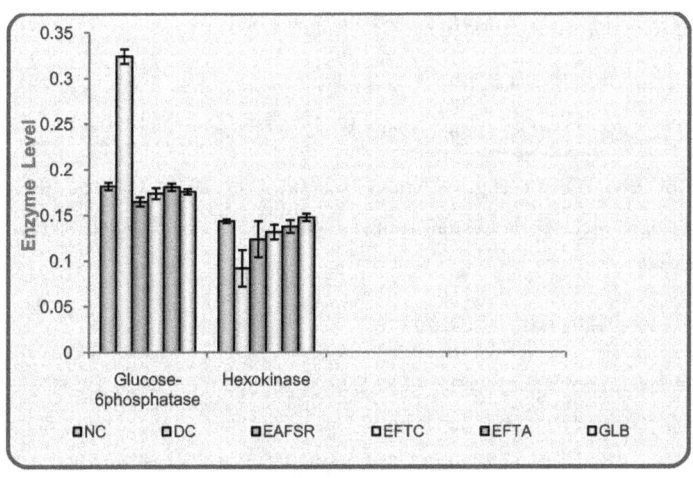

Graph 6.13 Effect on glucose-6-phosphatase and hexokinase in STZ induced diabetic rats.

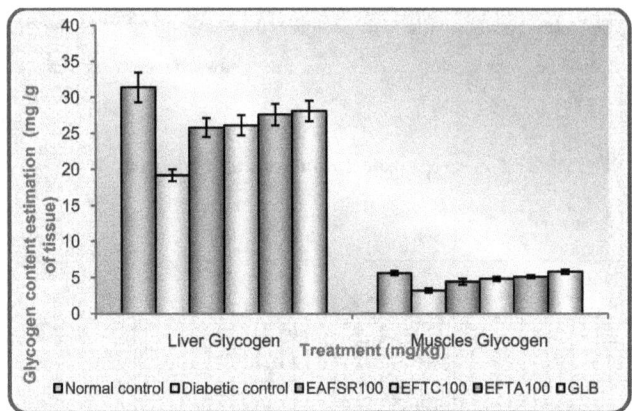

Graph 6.14 Effect of four weeks treatment of EAFSR, EFTC, EFTA and GLB glycogen level in diabetic rats

6.4.6 Effect on Hematological parameter in STZ induced diabetic rats

As per **Yakubu et al., 2007,** Hematological parameters give the information regarding homostasis of body. It explains blood related functions of plant fraction.

Estimation of RBC and WBC: as per **Mitruka and Rawnsley, 1977** RBC and WBC counted by the dilution of blood with diluting fluids in counting pipettes. haemocytometer was used for counting.

Estimation of heamoglobin (Hb) in blood:

Hemoglobin was determined using cynmeth-hemoglobin solution **(Carman, 1993).** Hb treated with potassium ferricyanide, potassium cyanide and potassium dihydrogenphosphate. The ferricyanide forms meth hemoglobin, which on reacting with cyanide converted into cyanmethemoglobin. The intensity of the colour formed is measured at 546 nm against blank.

The reagents used were from Diagnostic Kit. 0.02 ml of fresh whole blood was mixed with 5 ml of the cyanmeth reagent. At 546 nm optical density was measured after incubating at room temperature 5 min. The optical density of standard solution corresponding to 60 mg/dl hemoglobin at 546 nm

Table : 6.16 Effect on Hematological parameter in STZ induced diabetic rat

S.N.	Treatment (mg/kg)	Hb	Glycosylated Hb	RBC	WBC
1.	NC	14.20.±5.84	2.86±1.60	5.72±1.25	5.04±2.6
2.	DC	10.02±4.82**	7.34±2.50**	4.20±2.10**	3.24±1.2**
	EFSR	11.28±6.48**	6.24±1.66**	4.12±2.10**	3.4±2.34**
3.	EFTC	13.10±3.20*	4.70±2.84*	4.70±2.68*	4.65 ±2.2*
4.	EFTA	13.02±6.30*	4.00±2.06*	5.26±3.26*	4.68±2.20*
	GLB	14.02±5.14*	4.25±1.20*	5.32±0.26*	5.20±0.24*

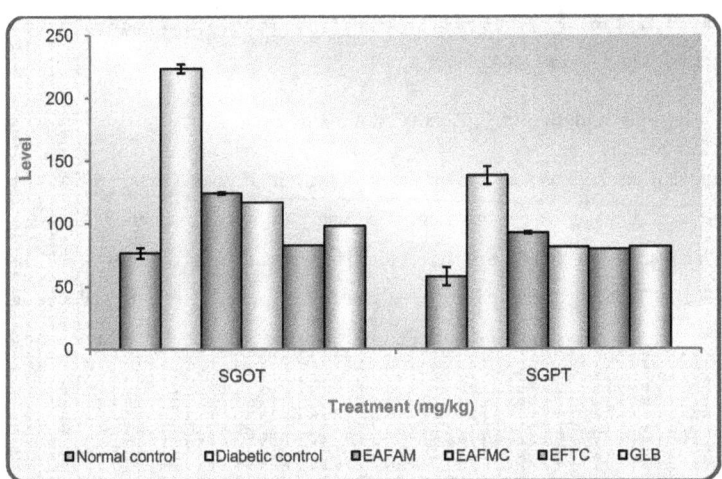

Graph 6.15 Effect on SGPT and SGOT in diabetic rats

ANTIDIABETIC EVALUATION OF PLANTS FRACTIONS

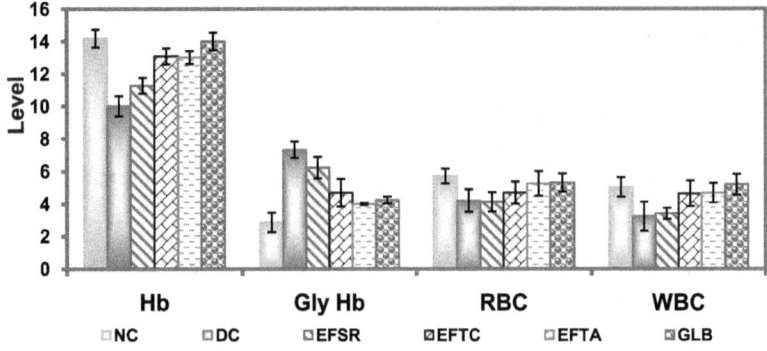

Graph 6.16: Effect on Hematological parameter in diabetic rats

6.4.7 Effect of four weeks repeated treatment of EAFSR, EFTC and EFTA on antioxidant activity in STZ induced diabetic rats

Effect on Lipid peroxidation in STZ induced diabetic rats

Free radicals are held responsible for the pathogenesis of several diseases like DM, atherosclerosis, cell damage, cancer, myocardial coronary thrombosis, hemolytc diseases, and immune diseases. The impact that free radicals make on lipids is known as lipid peroxidation (LP). The hyperglycemy in diabetes causes free radicals to be formed and the antioxidant system to become insufficient, thus increasing the oxidative stress (**Karasu,1999**).

Table 6.17 : Effects on MDA in streptozotocin-induced diabetic rats

S.No.	Treatment (mg/kg)	MDA

ANTIDIABETIC EVALUATION OF PLANTS FRACTIONS

1.	Normal control	2.68±0.28
2.	Diabetic control	8.40±0.65**
3.	EAFSR	5.16±0.32*
4.	EAFTC	4.54±0.31*
5.	EFTA	4.02±0.34*
6.	GLB	3.75±0.26*

6.4.8 Effect on Body and Organ Weight in streptozotocin induced diabetic rats:

Body and organ weight determinaed after four week. . Body and organ weight differences in between to diabetic control and diabetic treated rats were weighted on digital balance and tabulated (**Table 6.20,6.21;and Graph 6.17,6.18**).

Table 6.18: Effect on BWt in STZ-induced diabetic rats

S.No.	Treatment (mg/kg)	Body Weight (g)	
		Before treatment	After treatment
1.	Normal control	221.28±4.68	223.80±3.42
2.	Diabetic control	218.60±4.28	170.40±4.82
3.	EAFSR	220.24±5.10	182.66±4.24
4.	EFTC	213.64±6.82	186.00±5.8**
5.	EFTA	210.80±5.86	214.62±6.70**
6.	GLB (0.3mg)	216.20±4.74	218.46±5.04

Table 6.19 : Effects of fractions on body organ weight in streptozotocin-induced diabetic rats

S.No.	Treatment (mg/kg)	Body organ weight (g)		
		Liver	Pancreas	Kidney
1.	Normal control	1.72±0.24	0.38±0.02	0.62±0.03
2.	Diabetic control	5.10±0.45	0.41±0.03	0.66±0.01
3.	EAFSR	4.78±0.42	0.40±0.02	0.65±0.02
4.	EFTC	4.60±0.50	0.40±0.03	0.65±0.02
5.	EFTA	4.00±0.30	0.41±0.02	0.64±0.03
6.	GLB (0.3mg)	4.52±0.20	0.39±0.01	0.64±0.02

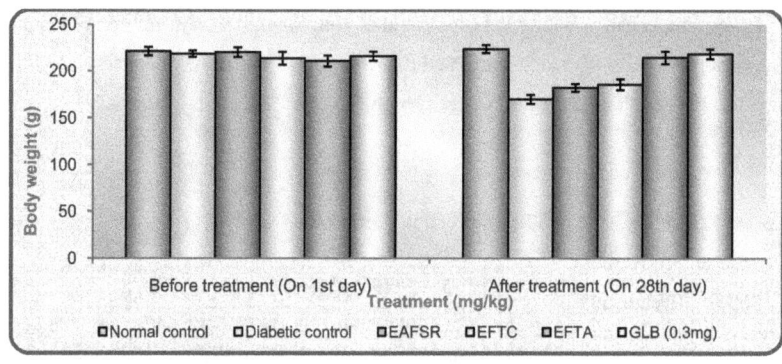

Graph 6.17 Effect of fractions on BWt in diabetic rats

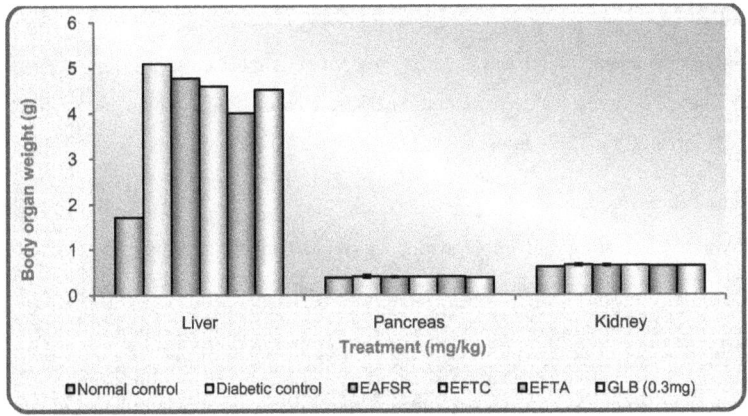

Graph 6.18 Effect of fractions on Body organ weight in diabetic rats

6.4.9 Histopathological observation

To evaluate the effect of consecutive four weeks repeated treatment of fractions in diabetic treated group of rats, histopathology of pancreas and liver tissues were done according to **Chakraborty and Chakraborty, 1998.**

Histopathological studies:

Histopathology of pancreas and liver of rats were carried out by method of **Chakraborty and Chakraborty, 1998**

(A) Fixation

Fixatives are agents which are used to preserve cells most closely to the original form in the body. Fixatives act by denaturation of proteins of tissues. small pieces were fixed in 10% formalin for 12-24 hours.

(B) Tissue Processing

Dehydration, clearing and impregnation is involved in tissue prossesing.Sections were prepared for cutting by embedding in paraffin wax that allowed the section to be cut.

(C) Blocking

L–blocks or l-moulds were used to prepare blocks. By simple manipulation of 2L-blocks, the size was altered as per the need of the tissue. The piece of tissue was kept in block and filled with molten wax.

(D) Section cutting

The tissue blocks were fastened to metal object holder when trimming them to acceptable size. A smear of egg albumen was ready and dirty on to the slide and dried. The tissue section of the 7μm thickness was cut with the assistance of scientific instrument Rotating Microtome. The tissue sections were placed on slide and drop on water so sections were floated in water on slide between 55-60°C, drained off and slides dried on hot plate at regarding 50°C for thirty min.

(E) Staining of sections

staining series followed as in **table 6.22** follows:

Table 6.22 staining series for Histopathology of pancreas and liver of rats

Down grade	Time (min)
Xylene	5
Absolute alcohol	5
Alcohol (90%)	5
Alcohol (70%)	5

Alcohol (50%)	5
Alcohol (30%)	5
Distilled water	5
Hematoxyline	10
Distilled water	10
Alcohol (30%)	5
Alcohol (50%)	5
Alcohol (70%)	5
Eosin	10
Alcohol (70%)	5
Alcohol (90%)	5
Absolute alcohol	5
Xylene	5

After passing from staining series cover with cover slip and the slides were observed under a compound microscope and photomicrographs were taken (photomicrograph6.1 and 6.2)

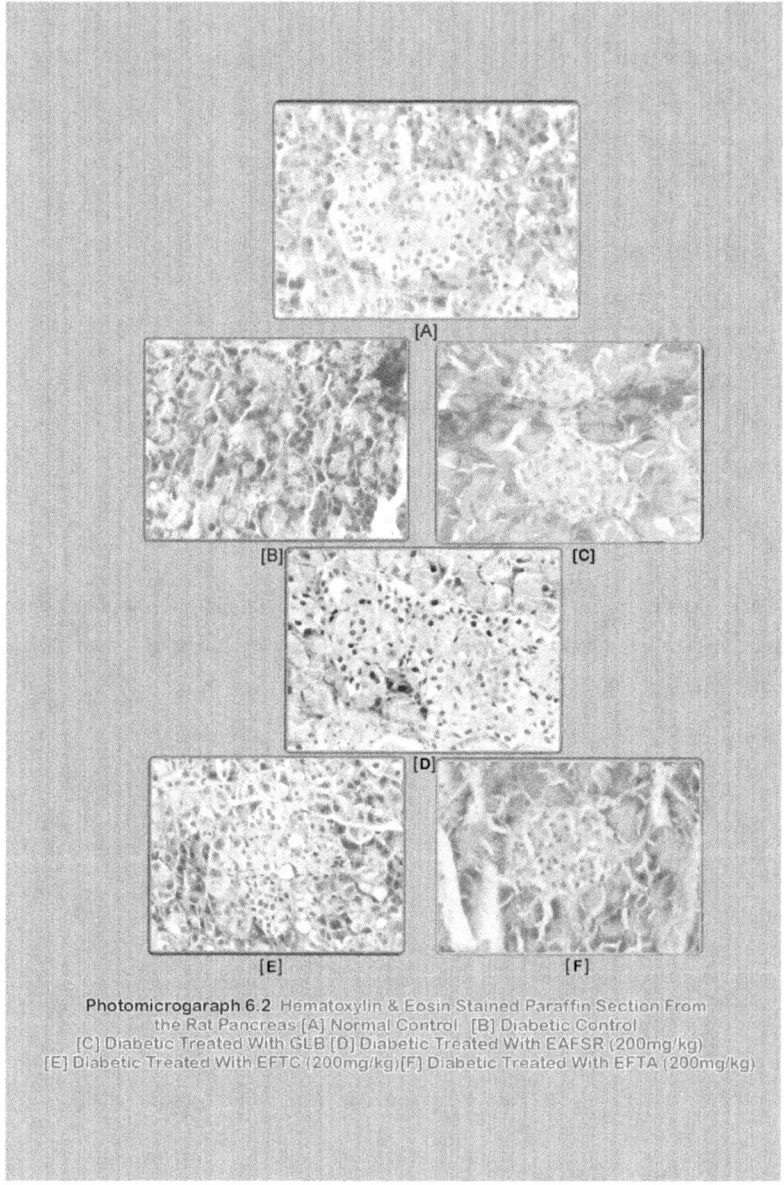

Photomicrogaraph 6.2 Hematoxylin & Eosin Stained Paraffin Section From the Rat Pancreas [A] Normal Control [B] Diabetic Control [C] Diabetic Treated With GLB [D] Diabetic Treated With EAFSR (200mg/kg) [E] Diabetic Treated With EFTC (200mg/kg) [F] Diabetic Treated With EFTA (200mg/kg)

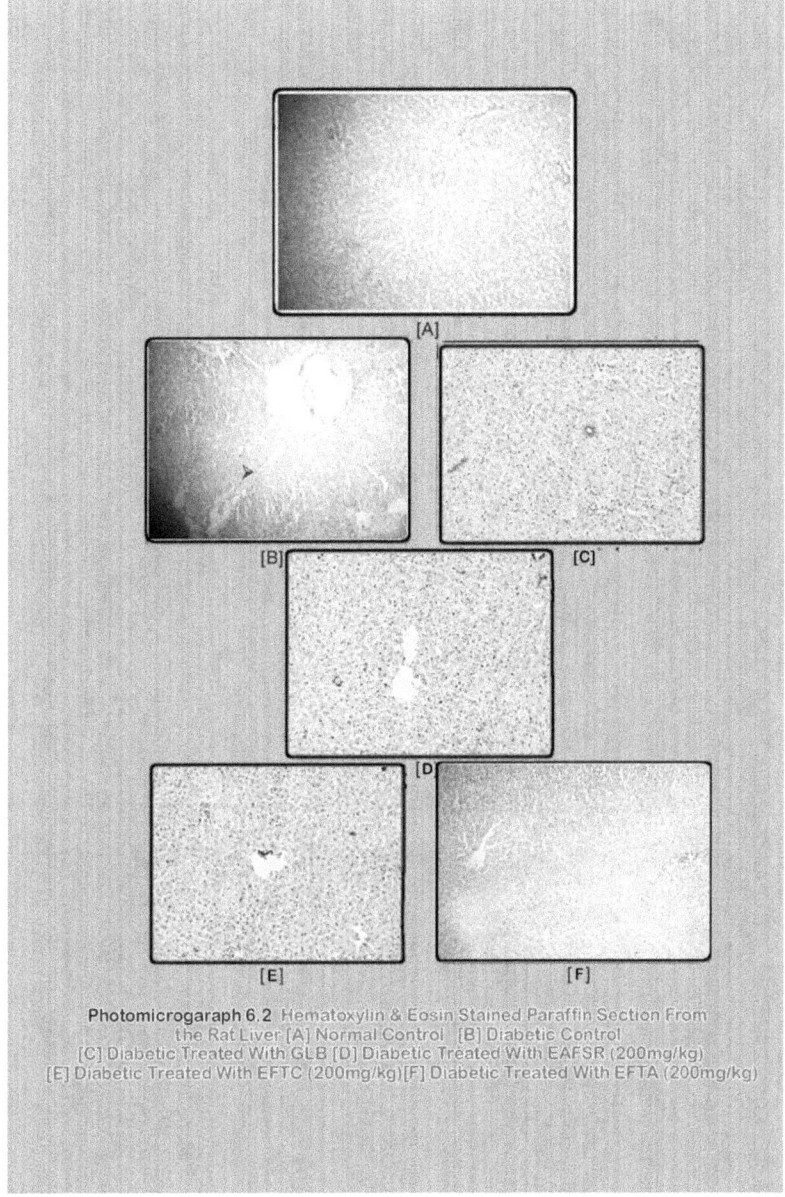

Photomicrogaraph 6.2 Hematoxylin & Eosin Stained Paraffin Section From the Rat Liver [A] Normal Control [B] Diabetic Control [C] Diabetic Treated With GLB [D] Diabetic Treated With EAFSR (200mg/kg) [E] Diabetic Treated With EFTC (200mg/kg) [F] Diabetic Treated With EFTA (200mg/kg)

FORMULATION DEVELOPMENT

7.1 DEVELOPMENT OF A STANDARDIZED FORMULATION

Herbs or herbal powders can be used as such if they have sufficient potency to exhibit medicinal action desired. If the herb is not potent enough to show the medicinal action with the maximum practical dose possible, then the medicinal properties can be potentiated by means of extract or fraction preparation. It was decided to convert selected plants fractions, which have antidiabetic property, into tablets.

7.2 TABLET FORMULATION

Because tablets are solid unit dosage forms having least content variability and suitable for large-scale production **(Lachman, 1987)**.

Therefore, it was decided to prepare tablets using spray dried powder of individual drug is more potent than its corresponding extract. It is also convenient and easy to prepare spray dried powder and have less chances of contamination or adulteration because it requires less no. of steps to prepare it, in comparison to extracts. Therefore, the spray dried powder of each plant material was selected to prepare the tablets.

7.3 CHARACTERIZATION OF SPRAY DRIED POWDER:

Drying of extracts is achieved by different conventional methods including tray drying, vacuum drying, spray drying and freeze drying. Ideal method of drying for herbal extract would be that which takes minimum period at a minimum temperature, with a minimum cost and still have a maximum cgygy ield and is capable of handling large quantities of extract. Freeze dried and spray dried extracts have an advantage of minimum thermal degradation. Spray drying has an advantage of fast drying with minimum period of exposure to drying temperature.

In the preparation of formulation, the spray-dried powder of each drug was studied and characterized as follows:

7.3.1 Organoleptic Characterization

The spray-dried powders of selected drug were properly characterized for their appearance, color, taste and odor **(Table 7.1)**.

FORMULATION DEVELOPMENT

Table 7.1 : Organoleptic characterization of spray dried powder of fraction of *S. rebaudiana*, *T. cordifolia* and *T. aestivum*

S.No.	Parameter	S. rebaudiana	T. cordifolia	T. aestivum
1.	Appearance	Powder	Powder	Powder
2.	Colour	Dark green	Dark Brown	Dark Brown
3.	Taste	Intense- sweet	Bitter	Bitter
4.	Odour	Sweetish	Characteristic	Characteristic

7.3.2 Ash Values :

Ash values for spray dried powder was estimated as per the procedure described for crude drugs. Results are tabulated as **Table 7.2**.

Table7.2: Ash values of spray dried powder of fractions

S.No.	Parameter	Total ash % w/w	Acid insoluble ash % w/w	Water soluble ash % w/w
1.	S. rebaudiana	7.5±0.4	0.018 ± 0.002	1.85 ± 0.06
2.	T. cordifolia	8.30 ± 0.52	0.026 ± 0.004	1.42 ± 0.07
3.	T. aestivum	6.86 ± 0.48	0.042 ± 0.008	0.68± 0.07

7.3.3 Moisture Pick up Values

Moisture pick up nature of any drug is one of the most important parameter in determining the method to be used for the preparation of tablet formulation and the excipients to be used in the formulation.

With the aim of preparation of tablet formulation from spray dried powder, their moisture pick up value was determined by keeping the powder in stability chambers at three different conditions of temperature and humidity.

Procedure:

Approximately 1 g of the spray dried powder was accurately weighed in three weighing bottles. The bottles were placed in 3 different stability chambers fixed at different temperature and humidity conditions. First chamber was fixed at 25°C temp. and 40%

relative humidity, second chamber was at 30°C temp. and 60% RH and third chamber at 40°C temp. and 75% RH. After one week, the samples were withdrawn from the chambers and again weighed and difference in their weight was calculated and percent moisture pick up value were calculated by comparing with their previous weight. The results are shown in **table 7.3** and the values are the average of three readings.

Table 7.3 : Percent moisture pick up by spray dried powder of fraction of *S. rebaudiana*, *T. cordifolia* and *T. aestivum* at different temperature and humidity conditions

Powder	% moisture pick up		
	25°C, 40% RH	30°C, 60% RH	40°C, 75% RH
S. rebaudiana	4.78 ± 0.38	6.40 ± 0.44	7.62 ± 0.52
T. cordifolia	5.34 ± 0.56	6.72 ± 0.52	8.34 ± 0.66
T. aestivum	5.21 ± 0.45	6.52 ± 0.50	7.30 ± 0.62

7.3.4 pH of 1% Dispersion

The acidic or alkaline nature of the spray dried powder of *S. rebaudiana*, *T. cordifolia* and *T. aestivum* was determined by preparing 1% mixture of these powder in distilled water. For this purpose, approximately 500 mg of the spray dried powder homogenized in 50 mL of DW. After half an hour, shaken and by using pH meter, pH was determined.

Table 7.4 : pH of 1% dispersion of fraction of *S. rebaudiana*, *T. cordifolia* and *T. aestivum* in water

S.No.	Spray dried powders	pH of 1%
1.	S. rebaudiana	7.8±0.2
2.	T. cordifolia	7.6±0.2
3.	T. aestivum	8.4±0.1

FORMULATION DEVELOPMENT

7.3.5 Bulk Density and Tap Density

The bulk density of the powder is usually it's weight or mass, in a specified volume.

Tap density of a powder is it's maximum packing density achieved under the externally applied forces.

Experimental:

To determine the bulk density of the spray dried powder, 20g powder of bioactive fraction of *S. rebaudiana, T. cordifolia* and *T. aestivum* was accurately weighed and transferred in a 100 ml measuring cylinder. The volume occupied by 20g of powder was note down and bulk density was calculated by using formula given.

For estimation of tap density of powder, the measuring cylinder containing 20g powder, was tapped 50 times on Electrolab Tap Density Tester. After 50 taps, the volume occupied by powder was note down and the tap density calculated by the given formula.

$$\text{Bulk Density} = \frac{\text{Weight of sample}}{\text{Volume of sample}}$$

$$\text{Tap Density} = \frac{\text{Weight of sample}}{\text{Volume of sample after 50 taps}}$$

Table 7.5 : Bulk and tap density of fraction of *S. rebaudiana, T. cordifolia* and *T. aestivum*

S.No.	Drugs	Bulk density	Tap density
1.	*S. rebaudiana*	0.36 mg/ml	0.425 mg/ml
2.	*T. cordifolia*	0.42 mg/mL	0.510 mg/mL
3.	*T. aestivum*	0.38 mg/mL	0.462 mg/mL

7.4 FORMULATION RECOMMENDATION

On the idea of preformulation studies (characterization of spray dried powder), it had been concluded that the tablets should be prepared by direct compression technique, because it is best for small-scale preparations.

Tablets were punched using hand rotating single punch machine. Microcrystalline cellulose (PH 101), was used because at 40°C temp. and 75% relative humidity, powder is picking up about 8% moisture, which indicates the hygroscopic nature of powder and MCC is non-hygroscopic, diluent additionally it has good binding properties also. Pregelatinized starch (PGS) was also taken **(Sworbrick et al., 1990 and Omray and Omrey, 1986)**.

The spray dried powder of fraction and different ingredients for every formula were weighed, mixed and versed sieve no.80 singly. Magnesium stearate used as a <u>diluent</u> and lubricants. All the materials were mixed along except Talc and Magnesium stearate were processed during a pestle and mortar and passed once more through sieve no.18. The materials were mixed with the binder resolution, that was further very {little} by little. Then Talc and Magnesium stearate were mixed in it. Tablets were punched victimization hand rotating single punch machine. The punching machine was cleansed properly. The punching machine was adjusted for the desired weight (per tablet) and hardness employing a tiny amount of the mix. when attaining the desired pill parameter, the full mix was punched into tablets **(Chaowalit et al, 2014 Manisha et al,2013)**.

The blend was compressed into tablets. Talc as lubricant and magnesium stearate as glidant. Their quantity was decided after various combinations of these ingredients, which gave the good flow at hopper and not causing the problem of capping, lamination or sticking. For formulations of tablet; talc as a lubricant and diluent was added which also tend to absorbs insignificant amount of moisture at 25°C and relative humidities up to about 90% and accelerates flow properties of powder. The tablets of fraction of *S. rebaudiana*, *T. cordifolia* and *T. aestivum* was incorporated in each prepared tablets amounting 250 mg of dose individually and named as **StevioTab, TinoTab** and **TriTab** respectively. **(Table 7.6, 7.7, 7.8)**.

FORMULATION DEVELOPMENT

Table 7.6 : Formulation of StivoTab tablet from *S. rebaudiana*

S.No.	Ingredient	Weight/Tablet
1.	Spray dried powder of *S. rebaudiana*	100
2.	Microcrystalline cellulose	100
3.	Pre gelatinized starch	25
4.	Magnesium stearate	15
5.	Talc	10

Table 7.7 : Formulation of TinoTab tablet from *T. cordifolia*

S.No.	Ingredient	Weight/ Tablet
1.	Spray dried powder of *T. cordifolia*	100
2.	Microcrystalline cellulose	100
3.	Pre gelatinized starch	25
4.	Magnesium stearate	15
5.	Talc	10

Table 7.8 : Formulation of TriTab tablet from *T. aestivum*

S.No.	Ingredient	Weight/Tablet
1.	Spray dried powder of *T. aestivum*	100
2.	Microcrystalline cellulose	100
3.	Pre gelatinized starch	25
4.	Magnesium stearate	15
5.	Talc	10

FORMULATION DEVELOPMENT

Drug excipients compatibility studies

There was no interaction between fractions and excipients selected for formulation. There is absence of any incompatibility under normal storage conditions in physical mixture.

7.5 EVALUATION OF PREPARED TABLETS

The prepared tablets of *S. rebaudiana*, *T. cordifolia* and *T. aestivum* were subjected for the following evaluation tests **(Indian Pharmacopoeia, 1996; Lachman *et al.*, 1987)**

- Weight Variation
- Hardness
- Friability
- Disintegration time
- Dissolution time
- Tablet assay for Drug Content By HPLC

7.5.1 Weight Variation Study

It was done to ensure that a tablet must contains the proper amount of drug. According to Indian Pharmacopoeia it must be within the limit.

Procedure:

20 tablets of the prepared spray dried powder tablets were weighed individually and their average weight was calculated and compared with the weight of individual tablet and the percent weight variation was calculated. **(Table 7.9).**

Table 7.9 : Weight variation of prepared antdiabetic tablets

S.No.	*Drug*	Weight variation
1.	StevioTab	3.52%
2.	TinoTab	2.84%
3.	TriTab	3.10%

FORMULATION DEVELOPMENT

7.5.2 Hardness Study

The tablet hardness is the force required to break a tablet. It was done by the use Monsanto hardness tester and the values are shown in **Table 7.10**.

Table 7.10 : Hardness test study of prepared tablets

Formulation Code	Hardness (kg/cm^2)					
	T1	T2	T3	T4	T5	Mean
StevioTab	5.2	5.3	5.2	4.8	4.4	4.9
TinoTab	5.4	4.8	5.0	4	5.2	4.8
TriTab	5.0	4.5	5.1	4.6	5.1	4.9

7.5.3 Friability Study

It was done to measure of tablet strength.

Procedure:

Friability of the prepared tablets was determined by placing 10 pre weighed tablets in Vigo scientific Friability tester, which was then operated for 100 revolutions (25 rpm for 4 min). After 100 revolutions, the weight of 10 tablets was again determined and percent friability was calculated by comparing the initial weight of the 10 tablets. **(Table 7.11)**.

Table 7.11 : Friability of prepared tablets

S.No.	*Drug*	*Friability (%)*
1.	StevioTab	0.13%
2.	TinoTab	0.14%
3.	TriTab	0.12 %

7.5.4 Disintegration Time Study

Disintegration is a process in which the tablets are breakdown in smaller particles or granules. It was by determined using IP Disintegration Apparatus (Indian Pharmacopoeia, 1996). One tablet was placed in each tube. In a one litre beaker which contain water at 37°C±2°C, basket positioned in a manner that the tablets remained 25 cm below the surface of the liquid on their upward movement and descend not closer than 25 cm from the bottom of the beaker. The frequency of the disintegration assembly was 30 cycles/min. and the time taken to pass the all disintegrated particles through 10-mesh screen was recorded and the values are shown **(Table 7.12)**.

For most tablets, the first important step toward solution is breakdown of the tablet into smaller particles or granules, a process known as disintegration. Disintegration time of the prepared tablets was determined using IP Disintegration Apparatus (Indian Pharmacopoeia, 1996) by placing one tablet in each tube and the basket was positioned in a one litre beaker of water at 37°C±2°C such that the tablets remained 25 cm below the surface of the liquid on their upward movement and descend not closer than 25 cm from the bottom of the beaker. The frequency of the disintegration assembly was 30 cycles/min. and the time taken to pass the all disintegrated particles through 10-mesh screen was recorded and the values are shown **(Table 7.12)**.

Table 7.12: Disintegration time study of prepared tablets

Formulation code	Disintegration time (min.)					
	T1	T2	T3	T4	T5	Mean
StevioTab	32.2	30.8	26.2	28.5	31.0	29.74
TinoTab	32.3	35.6	31.5	30.5	32.8	32.54
TriTab	30.2	32.6	34.2	28.4	26.5	30.38

7.5.5 Dissolution Time Study

The original rational for using tablet disintegration test was the fact that as the tablet break down into small particles, must be related to the bioavailability of the drug to the body. The rate of dissolution is related to the efficacy of the product. Therefore an evaluation as the whether or not a tablet releases its drug content were placed in the environment of the gastrointestinal tract is often fundamental concern to tablet formulator.

Procedure:

The dissolution time of the prepared tablets was determined by placing the tablet in the basket type dissolution apparatus. The basket was immersed in 0.1N HCl. The mortar was adjusting for 50 rpm and samples were withdrawn at 15, 30, 45 and 60 minutes interval and the amount of drug in solution was determined with the help of marker compound by HPLC. and results are tabulated **(Table 7.13).**

Table 7.13 : Dissolution time study of of prepared tablets at different time intervals

Time (minutes)	% dissolution of active constituents/markers		
	StevioTab	TinoTab	Tritab
	Stevioside	Berberine	Quercetin
15	30.24	32.20	29.80
30	62.10	58.98	44.82
45	81.56	78.00	77.64
60	90.48	95.24	92.25
120	98.79	98.98	99.54

7.6 Quantification Of Stevioside, Berberine And Quercetin In Steviotab, Tinotab And Tritab By HPLCMethod

Stevioside, Berberine and Quercetin were quantified in StevioTab, TinoTab and TriTab tablets for evaluating the content uniformity in terms of concentration of marker components.

FORMULATION DEVELOPMENT

Preparation of standard solution:

Accurately weighed about 10 mg of each standard compound dissolved in small quantity of ethanol and made up the volume 10 mL with ethanol in volumetric flask.

Preparation of sample solution:

Ten tablets of each (StevioTab, TinoTab and TriTab) were taken, powdered, dissolved in 100 mL ethanol. Sample and standard were filtered through 0.15 μm filter paper, and transferred to HPLC vial and placed inside the HPLC auto sampler chamber. The system was standardized for the HPLC instrument and the analysis was accomplished.

Procedure:

HPLC procedure for the estimation of Stevioside, Berberine and Quercetin in StevioTab, TinoTab and TriTab tablets was used as per the previous section 3.7.2 of the Chapter 3rd and results were recorded **(Table 7.14, 7.15 and 7.16).**

The amount of Stevioside present in 10 μl amount of Stevio**Tab** is 0.2642μg; therefore tablet (100 mg of fraction)will comprised 2642μg of Stevioside.

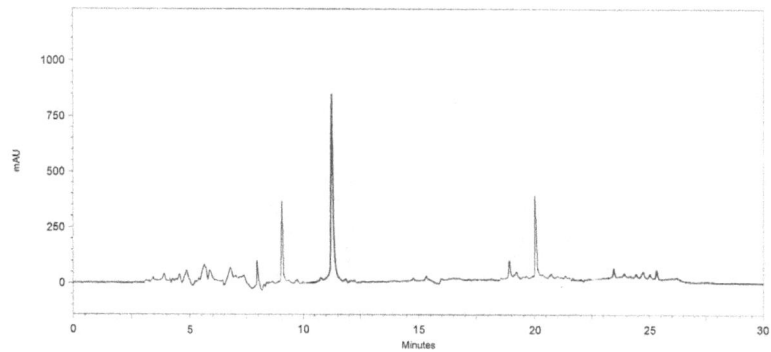

Peak	RT	Area	Height
1	4.631	61334	484650

Fig. 7.1 : HPLC chromatogram of StevioTab

FORMULATION DEVELOPMENT

Table 7.14 : Estimation of Stevioside in Stevio Tab tablet by HPLC

Replicate	Sample area	Stevioside (µg)
1	61365	0.2651
2	61340	0.2644
3	61297	0.2631
Average	61334	0.2642

The amount of Berberine present in 10 µl amount of TinoTab is 0.021µg, therefore 250 mg of tablet (100 mg of fraction) was found to be 282.3 µg of Berberine. The HPLC chromatogram of TinoTab is shown in **Figure 7.2**.

Table 7.15: Estimation of Berberine in TinoTab tablet by HPLC

Replicate	Sample area	Berberine (µg)
1	1146087	0.2830
2	1899012	0.2818
3	11390753	0.2845
Average	14435852	0.2832

FORMULATION DEVELOPMENT

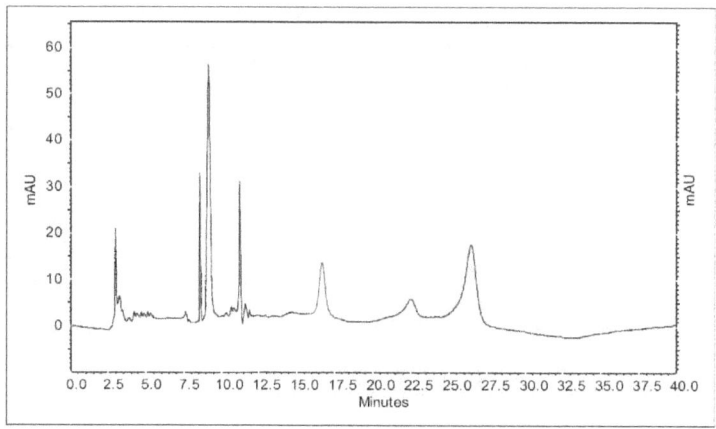

Peak	RT	Area	Height
1	8.35	1899012	629463

Fig. 7.2 : HPLC chromatogram of TinoTab

Estimation of Quercetin in TriTab

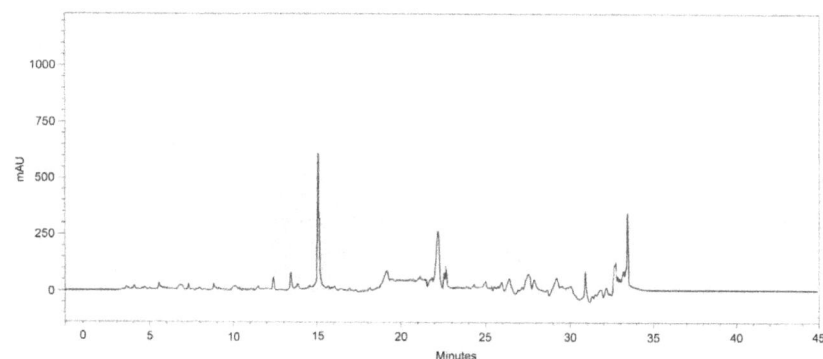

Peak	RT	Area	Height
1	15.1	61961	391460

Fig. 7.3 : HPLC chromatogram of TriTab

Table 7.16: Estimation of Quercetin in TriTab tablet by HPLC

Replicate	Sample area	Quercetin (µg)
1	62008	0.6254
2	61745	0.6182
3	62131	0.6288
Average	61961	0.6241

The amount of Quercetin present in 10 µl amount of TriTab is 0.6241, therefore 250 mg of tablet (100 mg of fraction) was found to be 6241µg of Quercetin. The HPLC chromatogram of TriTab is shown in Figure 7.3.

7.7 ACCELERATED STABILITY STUDIES OF PREPARED TABLETS

The Polyherbal antidiabetic formulation developed needs to be checked for its stability, hence a study is undertaken to subject the tablet formulation to Accelerated stability studies. The prepared tablets (StevioTab, TinoTab and TriTab) were analysed for color, mottling, weight variation, hardness and quantification of the marker compound.

Stability studies

The tablet formulation kept in stability chamber at 40°C and 75% RH (relative humidity) for six month after packing in aluminium foil.

One packet of 30 gms of Silica gel was kept inside the tablet container to absorb moisture and packed with cotton on the mouth and then closed with a cap. For stability study parameters, tablets were checked for six months. The results were tabulated as follows **(Table 7.17, 7.18,7.19and 7.20).**

Table 7.17: Stability studies of prepared antidiabetic tablets

Tablet	Colour	Hardness (Kg/cm2)	Friability (%)	Disintegration time (min.)	Weight variation (%)
StevioTab	No distinct Change	NMT 5	NMT 1.0%	NMT 40	No distinct change
TinoTab	No distinct Change	NMT 6	NMT 1.0%	NMT 40	No distinct Change
TriTab	No distinct Change	NMT 5	NMT 1.0%	NMT 35	No distinct Change

NMT : Not More Than

Table 7.18 : Quantitation of Stevioside in StevioTab tablet by HPLC

Replicate	Stevioside (µg/tablet) (0 month)	Stevioside (µg/tablet) (3 months)	Stevioside (µg/tablet) (6 months)
1.	0.035	0.035	0.035
2.	0.037	0.036	0.036
3.	0.036	0.035	0.035
Average	0.036±0.0	0.035± 0.00	0.035± 0.00

FORMULATION DEVELOPMENT

Table 7.19 : Quantitation of Berberine in TinoTab tablet by HPLC

Replicate	Berberine (µg /tablet) (0 month)	Berberine (µg /tablet) (3 months)	Berberine (µg /tablet) (6 months)
1.	0.025	0.024	0.024
2.	0.024	0.024	0.023
3.	0.025	0.024	0.024
Average	0.024±0.0	0.024± 0.00	0.023± 0.00

Table 7.20 : Quantitation of Quercetin in TriTab tablet by HPLC

Replicate	Quercetin (µg/tablet) (0 month)	Quercetin (µg/tablet) (3 months)	Quercetin (µg/tablet) (6 months)
1.	0.029	0.028	0.028
2.	0.029	0.029	0.029
3.	0.030	0.028	0.028
Average	0.029	0.028	0.028

COMPARISION OF FORMULATIONS

Divya madhunashini vati is effective diabetes It decrease BG, increases insulin secretion. It's regular use improves health of diabetic person and restore the negative impact of diabetes in individual. It contains mainly Shilajit, ashwagandha, gurmar and giloy along with some other herbs.

A study was conducted to compare developed formulation i.e. **StevioTab, TinoTab** and **TriTab** with **Madhunashini Vati** which is well stablished antidiabetic herbomineral formulation, to evaluate the efficacy of **StevioTab, TinoTab** and **TriTab**. It administered in rats orally by suspending in DW using orogastric tube at a dose of 1 g/kg. The ingestable volume was constant i.e. 5 ml/kg. only vehicle was given orally to control animals

8.1 BLOOD GLUCOSE DETERMINATION IN STREPTOZOTOCIN-INDUCED DIABETIC RATS

Chronic antidiabetic activity of formulations i.e. **StevioTab, TinoTab, TriTab, Madhunashini Vati** and GLB determined in STZ-induced diabetic rats. After two hours of last treatment, BG was determined **(Table 8.1; Graph 8.1).**

Table 8.1 : Effects of four weeks administration of StevioTab, TinoTab, TriTab and Madhunashini Vati on blood glucose level in streptozotocin induced diabetic rats.

S.No.	Treatment (mg/kg)	Blood glucose conc.	
		Blood glucose Before Treated	Blood glucose After Treated
1.	Normal control	84.65±4.01	83.98±3.44
2.	Diabetic control	280.62±6.21	305.22±7.52**
3.	StevioTab	282.50±6.30	117.30±4.85*
4.	TinoTab	288.72±5.45	105.88±5.62*
5.	TriTab	285.26±4.08	122.56±6.46*
6	Madhunashini Vati	290.16±7.12	102.40±5.01*
7.	GLB	284.80±6.46	108.20±4.76*

OGTT was carried out to ascertain the activity of formulations and GLB in the presence of high glucose load. Administered 1.5 g/kg body wt of glucose, orally to overnight fasted animals. Standard group received glibenclamide, treated groups received different fractions, control groups received only vehicle, before the administration of glucose. B. G was estimated from 30 min to 2h. **(Table 8.2; Graph 8.2).**

Table 8.2 : Effect of four weeks repeated treatment of formulations on OGTT in streptozotocin-induced diabetic rats

S. No.	Treatment (mg/kg)	Blood glucose (mg/dl)			
		0 h (FBG)	1/2 h	1 h	2 h
1.	Normal control	87.80±4.56	162.24±5.30	139.48±5.22	90.10±4.10
2.	Diabetic control	294.40±8.22	398.20±9.62**	371.44±8.30**	368.20±9.50**
3.	StevioTab	148.48±4.74	272.70±8.12*	250.24±7.12*	170.65±8.56*
4.	TinoTab	138.00±5.02	260.47±7.42*	212.10±5.84*	162.66±7.52*
5.	TriTab	150.40±4.56	286.20±7.18*	251.12±6.36*	182.30±8.36*
6	Madhunashini Vati	132.30±5.90	235.24±7.24*	192.40±6.30*	148.20±9.42*
7.	GLB	124.30±6.10	204.15±7.36*	172.40±3.16*	150.28±6.02*

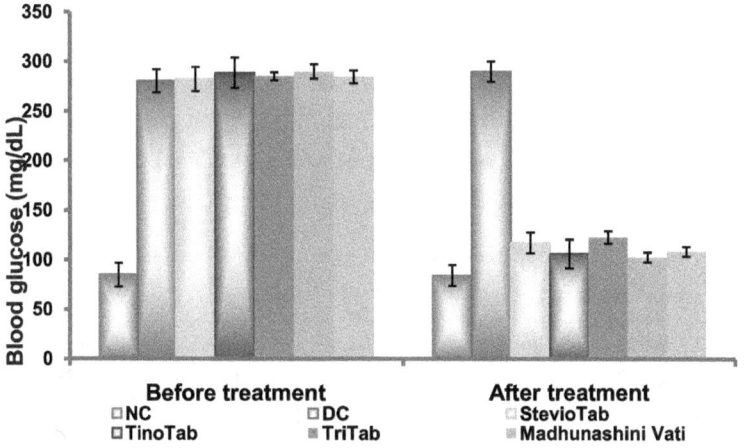

Graph 8.1 Effect of four weeks treatment of formulations on blood glucose in streptozotocin-induced diabetic rats

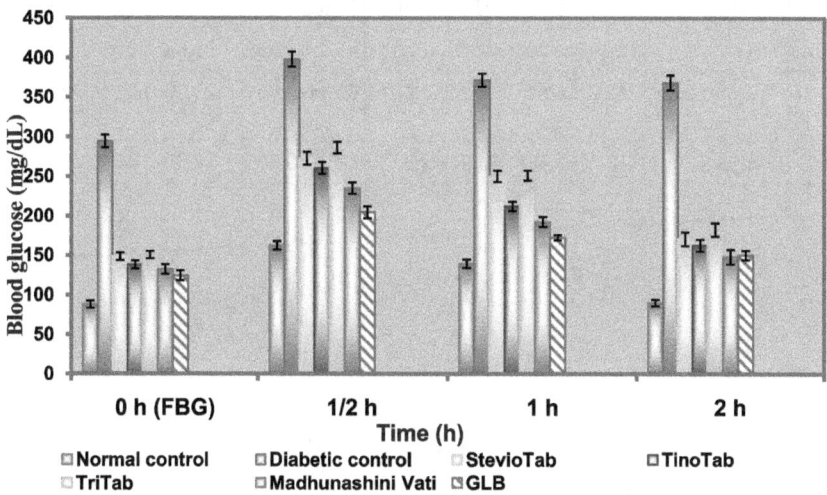

Graph 8.2 Effect of four weeks treatment of formulations on OGTT in streptozotocin-induced diabetic rats

8.2 EFFECT OF REPEATED DOSE TREATMENT OF FORMULATIONS ON LIPID PROFILE IN STREPTOZOTOCIN INDUCED DIABETIC RATS

Lipid profile (Total cholesterol, HDL, LDL, VLDL and TG) in serum were estimated as per protocol of availed kits (Tran Asia Bio Medical Limited, Mumbai, India). All the lipid profile estimation data were expressed in mg/dl **(Table 8.3; Graph 8.3).**

Table 8.3 : Effect of four weeks repeated treatment of formulations on lipid profile in streptozotocin-induced diabetic rats

S. No.	Treatment (mg/kg)	Cholesterol (mg/dl)	HDL (mg/dl)	LDL (mg/dl)	VLDL (mg/dl)	TG (mg/dl)
1.	Normal control	108.08±4.01	36.11±2.32	53.23± 3.02	28.34±1.21	135.88±6.80
2.	Diabetic control	179.26±3.98**	19.05±1.60**	125.40±7.42**	34.20±1.22**	205.80±7.40**
3.	StevioTab	122.16±4.80*	38.42±1.24*	57.72±3.50*	30.80±1.40*	138.40±6.12*
4.	TinoTab	118.24±5.02*	41.50±1.46*	70.62±3.86*	27.64±2.32*	132.24±5.62*
5.	TriTab	120.94±6.20*	38.21±1.80*	64.28±3.10*	32.08±1.20*	142.52±6.40*
6	Madhunashini Vati	115.22±6.84*	40.52±2.66*	62.34±3.00*	29.30±1.22*	132.22±5.06*
7.	GLB	112.32±3.44*	42.00±2.32*	48.74±3.10*	28.36±1.40*	133.64±4.40*

8.3 EFFECT OF REPEATED DOSE TREATMENT OF FORMULATIONS ON SGPT, SGOT AND LIPID PEROXIDATION IN STREPTOZOTOCIN INDUCED DIABETIC RATS

The blood plasma was analyzed for MDA, SGOT and SGPT using standard procedures in an Autoanalyzer. For this blood samples were taken in Eppendroff's tubes which already contain trisodium citrate solution, separated the plasma by centrifugation and stored in a refrigerator until analysis.

Table 8.4 : Effect of four weeks treatment of formulations on SGOT, SGPT and MDA in streptozotocin-induced diabetic rats

S.No.	Treatment (mg/kg)	SGOT	SGPT	MDA
1.	Normal control	78.2±3.1	60.4±3.1	2.76±0.26
2.	Diabetic control	239.4±7.4**	131.2±7.2**	8.78±0.71**
3.	StevioTab	115.1±4.5*	84.4±6.1*	3.34±0.36*
4.	TinoTab	98.6±5.4*	68.8±3.9*	3.20±0.28*
5.	TriTab	79.2±4.2*	73.8±6.4*	3.12±0.35*
6.	Madhunashini Vati	78.4±3.2*	74.2±5.8*	3.00±0.32*
7.	GLB	98.2±4.6*	80.4±6.2*	3.60±0.31*

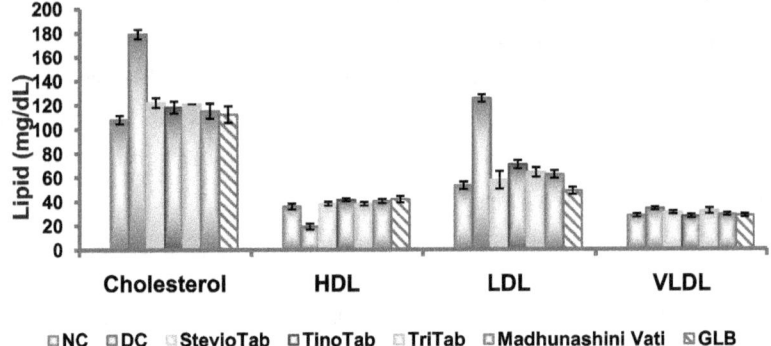

Graph 8.3: Effect of four weeks treatment of formulations on lipid profile in streptozotocin-induced diabetic rats

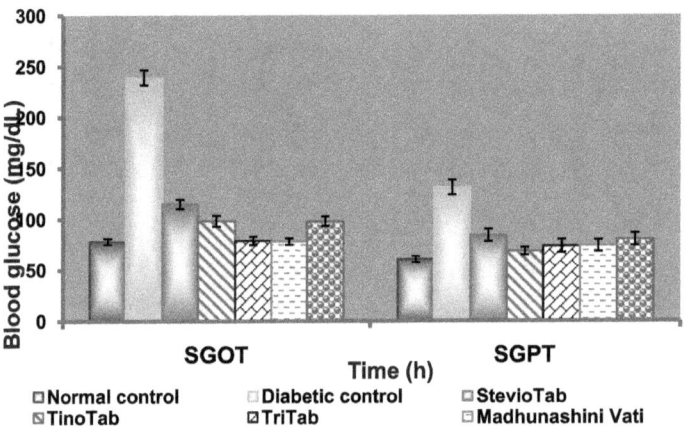

Graph 8.4: Effect of four weeks treatment of formulations on SGOT and SGPT in streptozotocin-induced diabetic rats

8.4 EFFECT OF FORMULATIONS ON BODY WEIGHT IN STREPTOZOTOCIN INDUCED DIABETIC RATS

In the present study, repeated dose treatment of formulations for four weeks were examined for body weight determination in streptozotocin-induced diabetic rats.

Table 8.5 : Effect of four weeks treatment of formulations on body weight in streptozotocin-induced diabetic rats

S.No.	Treatment (mg/kg)	Body weight (g)	
		Before treatment	After treatment
1.	Normal control	218.10±4.10	225.60±5.28
2.	Diabetic control	202.60±4.28	182.62±3.92**
3.	StevioTab	220.24±5.10	207.22±6.12*
4.	TinoTab	213.64±6.82	215.60±6.10*
5.	TriTab	212.40±4.92	212.12±5.46*
6	Madhunashini Vati	192.28±4.70	198.20±5.24*
7.	GLB	210.40±4.62	215.82±5.08*

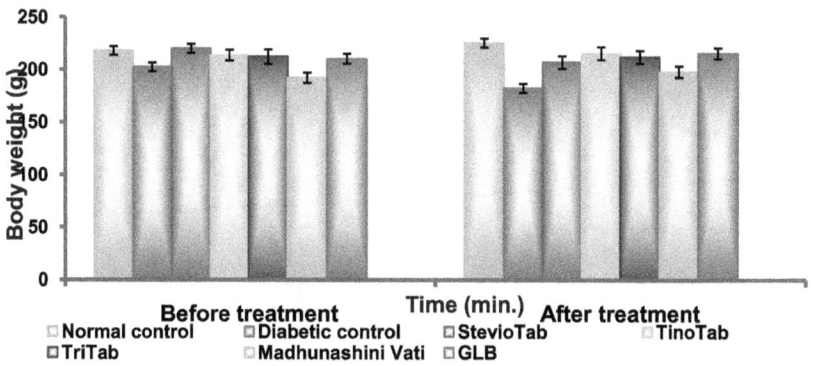

Graph 8.5: Effect of four weeks treatment of formulations on Body Weight in streptozotocin-induced diabetic rats

www.ingramcontent.com/pod-product-compliance
Lightning Source LLC
LaVergne TN
LVHW010215070526
838199LV00062B/4589